Joy Dowey Zonavetch

A History of Healing, A Future of Care

Saint Mary of Nazareth Hospital Center:
Celebrating a Century of Catholic Hospitality

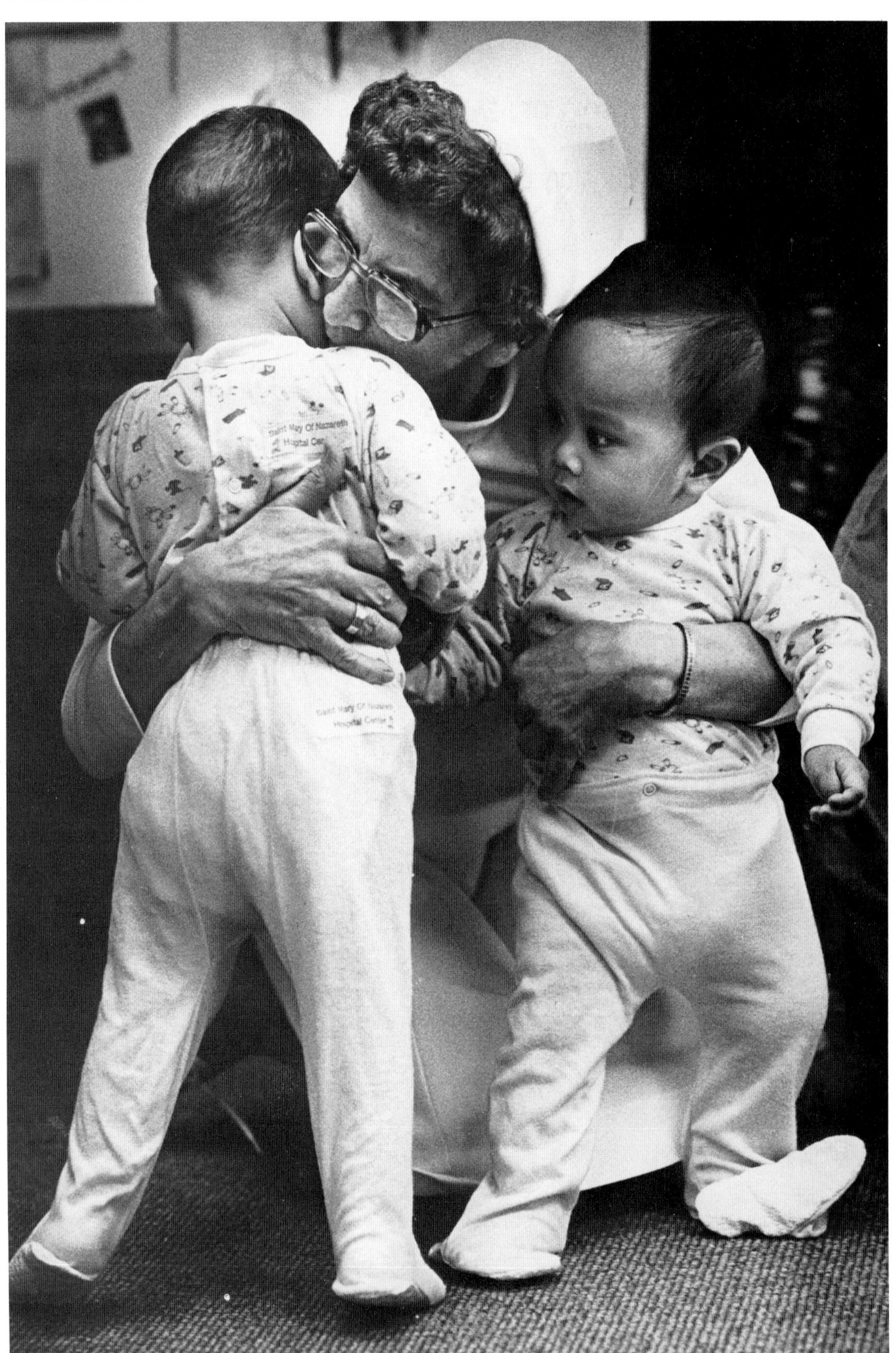
Saint Mary Of Nazareth

A HISTORY OF HEALING, A FUTURE OF CARE

Saint Mary of Nazareth Hospital Center:
Celebrating a Century of Catholic Hospitality

by

CHARLES W. SANFORD, JR.

Edited by

PHYLLIS PAVESE
and
RODNEY NELSON

C. WAYNE HAMILTON
Senior Historical Consultant

Heritage Publishers, Inc.
Flagstaff, Arizona

A HISTORY OF HEALING, A FUTURE OF CARE

Saint Mary of Nazareth Hospital Center:
Celebrating a Century of Catholic Hospitality

by Charles W. Sanford, Jr.

Edited by Phyllis Pavese and Rodney Nelson
C. Wayne Hamilton—Senior Historical Consultant
Designed by Vanessa Davisson

Heritage Publishers, Inc.
2700 Woodlands Boulevard, Suite 300
Flagstaff, Arizona 86001-7124
(602) 526-1129 (800) 972-8507

ISBN 929690-24-9
Library of Congress Cataloging Number 94-75721

Printed and bound in the United States of America

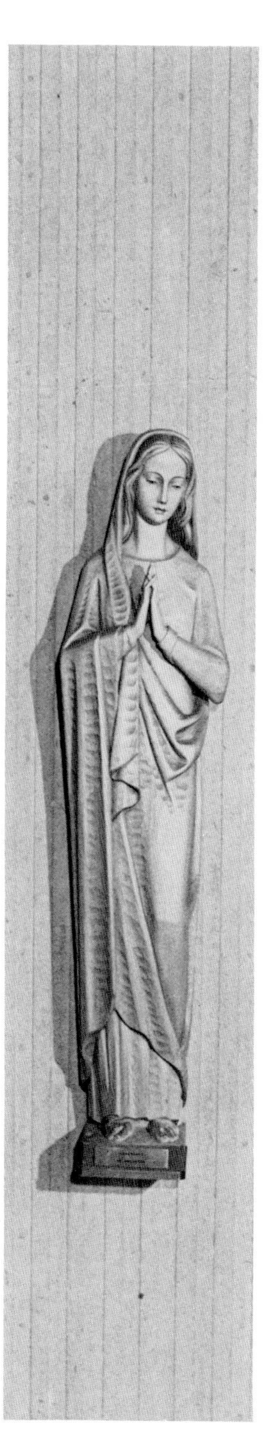

DEDICATION

To the past, for all that
we've learned...
To the present, for all that we are...
To the future, for all that we hope...

This centennial album is dedicated
to all the members of the
Saint Mary of Nazareth Hospital family...
Sisters, physicians, nurses, employees and
volunteers... past and present who
have given 100 years of love and caring
to the sick and suffering patients of this
institution and to the
Chicagoland community.

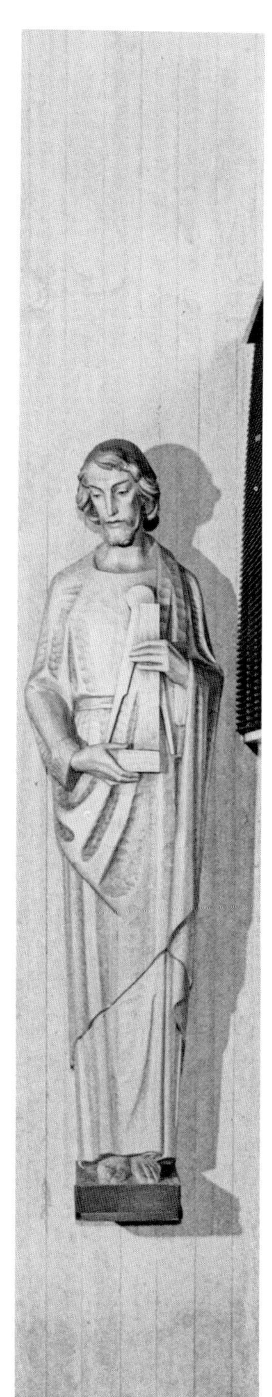

CONTENTS

FOREWORD

Many things have changed in our part of Chicago since 1894. Medical science has made progress that would have been unimaginable when our doors opened. Rudimentary medical procedures of a century ago have become sophisticated and complex. The newest emulation of the original 24-bed brownstone building is a 16-story healthcare center. We have seen the physical requirements of the hospital skyrocket, then smooth out, while the number of patients treated continues to rise.

That small group of Polish Sisters who led the way—members of the Congregation of Sisters of the Holy Family of Nazareth—now number 1,300 hospital employees, 270 doctors, 22 Sisters and an ever-growing league of kindred spirits, our loyal laity.

In many ways, the needs of our community haven't changed all that much over the past century. Human beings are much the same. They need good care cheerfully provided, decent wages to support their families, and the hope of a good tomorrow.

Many things about Saint Mary's will never change, and I think those are the most important. Our community of Sisters and our ministries are deeply dedicated to support for families, to serving those who need us most, to our provision of good care and to our emphasis on Christ-centered work.

Sister Stella Louise

Sister Stella Louise, CSFN
President and Chief Executive Officer
Saint Mary of Nazareth Hospital Center
February 1994

ACKNOWLEDGMENTS

This anniversary book is the result of the experience, work and devotion of so many people.

The extensive chronology written by Sister Mary Edith was an indispensable guide to Saint Mary's history.

The direction, insights and information provided by Sister Stella Louise, Wayne Hamilton and Joseph Boton have been essential.

The overall coordination, research, knowledge and day-to-day assistance of Phyllis Pavese has been critical to the success of this publication.

Our warmest thanks to Sister Bernadette for her help in identifying dozens of photographs, and to Sister Antonia for her contributions to the School of Nursing research.

Archivist Joseph Zurawski contributed much by his organization of the hospital archives.

The wonderful memories of all those who were interviewed for the book were delightful. Thank you for sharing them.

While we could not include every person, every fact and every memory, we have done our best to be accurate. We apologize for any inadvertent errors or omissions. Look for any additions in our next jubilee book!

Now, enjoy this story of Saint Mary's first 100 years...

SECRETARIAT OF STATE

FIRST SECTION - GENERAL AFFAIRS

FROM THE VATICAN,

No. 344933

February 25, 1994

Dear Mother Maria Teresa,

The Holy Father was pleased to learn that St. Mary of Nazareth Hospital Center in Chicago is commemorating the centenary of its foundation. He wishes me to convey his cordial good wishes and the assurance of his closeness in prayer.

His Holiness joins you and your Sisters in giving thanks to Almighty God for the apostolic zeal and charitable concern which prompted Blessed Mary of Jesus the Good Shepherd to establish a hospital destined to meet the medical and spiritual needs of the Polish immigrant community in Chicago. He prays that the present celebrations will be a source of inspiration and encouragement to the hospital administration and staff in their efforts to serve people of all ethnic backgrounds with love, patience and compassion. It is his particular hope that the Sisters of the Holy Family of Nazareth serving in the Hospital Center will dedicate themselves with renewed vigor to the apostolate of health care, bearing ever more joyful witness of their consecration as faithful disciples of Christ the Good Samaritan.

With these sentiments, the Holy Father willingly imparts his Apostolic Blessing to all those associated with St. Mary of Nazareth Hospital Center, invoking upon them grace and peace in the Lord.

Sincerely yours in Christ,

+G. B. Re
Substitute

Mother Maria Teresa Jasionowicz, C.S.F.N.
Superior General
Sisters of the Holy Family of Nazareth
Via Nazareth, 400
00166 Rome

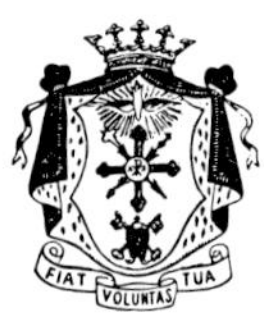

SUORE DELLA SACRA FAMIGLIA DI NAZARETH
CASA GENERALIZIA
VIA NAZARETH, 400 00166 ROMA, ITALIA

February 22, 1994

Dear Sister Stella Louise and St. Mary of Nazareth Hospital Center Community,

Every celebrated anniversary takes us back to the origins - marvelous origins - in this event the origins of St. Mary of Nazareth Hospital Center! The Gospel message of love, mercy and compassion experienced and dynamically lived by Blessed Mary of Jesus the Good Shepherd (Frances Siedliska) is implanted with trembling but decisive hands in Chicago! It is planted with great faith and with immense hope; faith in an everlasting love of God; hope in His word. Our Blessed Foundress heard God saying with impelling force: "Leave all and go out to them...in my name. I have chosen you as a visible sign and an effective messenger of my redeeming love for them. Do not be afraid; I will be with you. I will give you my spirit." (Jer. 1: 4-10 and Is. 6: 6-8)

The Congregation's first Constitutions echo these scriptural words: (Chapter 19)

Following the example of Christ Jesus who loved the poor and the suffering in a special manner...the sisters shall, out of love for their Divine Spouse, dedicate themselves to the service of the poor and the suffering with great compassion and kindness. In the poor and the suffering the sisters shall acknowledge the person of our Divine Lord, and for this reason they shall regard them with the greatest kindness and treat them with high respect and charity.

We celebrate a span of time -- 100 years -- 1894 to 1994 -- a century -- made of minutes, hours, days, months and years -- impregnated with that urging appeal addressed to our Mother Foundress and received by the Congregation as its special mission flowing from our charism, to spread the Kingdom of God's love.

In 1894 a small hospital opened. This little, humble seed planted with passion and with love-directed risk takes root, grows slowly, expands, flourishes, reaches the skies. Today St. Mary's magnificent structure with all the modern equipment that we contemplate with awe-full admiration, is a reflection of that interior force flowing from our charism with which the sisters responded to the calling of the Spirit and the crying needs of the people. What gave the Congregation the power to pierce through all the difficulties, lack of means, rejection? The love of God which burned in the heart of our Mother Foundress transmitted to her sisters the mission of compassionate love for the poorest of the poor - the homeless, sick, despairing, unwanted, the burdensome to society - the IMMIGRANTS. Gradually St. Mary's became a beacon calling and receiving the needy.

2.

When you look at St. Mary's, the structure itself will tell the story of love. Cooperating with the help of medical science to alleviate the distress of the sick, the sisters and those who minister there spread at the same time kindness and loving compassionate care for the whole person that not even the most sophisticated medical assistance could provide. The hospital has become a family center, a home, a shrine, a place where man feels more man, where his dignity is stressed and asserted, where the original features of similarity to the Trinity are restored to his body, soul and his whole being. (Gen. 1: 26-27, Wis. 2:23) It has become a place from which the Gospel message of Jesus' concern, compassion and mercy is proclaimed. It is a place where grace and nature are mobilized to serve man created in God's image and likeness.

We touch here the great mystery of the Incarnation. Mary, the Mother of Jesus, is at the beginning of this mystery. She gave human life to Jesus and stands in eternal vigilance over every life. As the Encyclical Redemptor Hominis states, "Christ accepting our human nature in a certain way united Himself with every man and thus gave to human life an immense dignity." (#8)

At St. Mary's, life is asserted and proclaimed more than ever before because today it is so dangerously menaced from its conception to its death. No race, culture, religion or conviction are excluded from St. Mary's care. The door of this hospital is opened to all. It has become an Ecumenical Center - par excellance. Our Congregation marked by the mystery of the Incarnation is of its essence ecumenical; ecumenism being a joyful and dynamic consequence of the deep understanding of the Incarnation.

May the Mother of God, Mary of Nazareth, the special patron of this hospital make you more and more aware of her motherhood which extends from the Incarnation of her first born to every birth of a human being. In Jesus she became the mother of all life. May she make you apostles, instruments and servants of divine goodness and mercy addressed to life.

I desire that this centennial be celebrated in a spirit of humble thanksgiving for the great deeds accomplished at St. Mary of Nazareth Hospital Center. May it continuously stand in the middle of other buildings as a luminous, courageous, vibrant, prophetical sign of life:

- of its venerated acceptance as an inviolable gift of God since its conception;
- of its affirmation in all its manifestations - healthy or disabled; and
- of its conservation through care and compassion to the last natural breath through love-invented means.

3.

Let St. Mary's be a glorious song of the living, soaring high with an uninterrupted praise for the source of LIFE and for all life. May it be a Magnificat, sung with Her who gave life to her first born and became the mother of all life. Let all generations, past, present and future call St. Mary's "Blessed" because in this place, God, rich in mercy, meets constantly with His beloved people. (Eph. 2: 4)

May God bless Sister Stella Louise, the hospital's dynamic and enthusiastic administrator, the sisters, doctors, staff and all who dedicate themselves to the patients at St. Mary's. Today Jesus thanks you and your predecessors for all the good deeds that were and are being accomplished here. He accepts all your services to others as done to Himself for "whatever you did to these little ones you did it to me." (Matt. 25: 40)

Looking at the past you must feel deep gratitude, pride and satisfaction in the tremendous growth and expansion of this hospital. Looking towards the future your hearts should be filled with hope and trust, for God will do great things for you measured according to your self surrendering love and trust. He who has begun this work in you and through you will accomplish it in His due time.

In this Year of the Family, you are challenged once again to respond to the repeated appeal of our Holy Father, John Paul II, to reach out to all families especially those whom society rejects. Today more than ever, the world is thirsting for divine mercy and you are called by your very charism to offer to the needy this marvelous water that restores health to soul and body.

The Congregation of the Sisters of the Holy Family of Nazareth, Associates, families, friends, and those to whom you minister join you today in singing an uninterrupted Magnificat for the great things God has accomplished through St. Mary of Nazareth Hospital Center since its humble beginnings to the present day.

With warmest congratulations,

M. Maria Teresa Jasionowicz

Mother Maria Teresa Jasionowicz, C.S.F.N.
Superior General

THE WHITE HOUSE

WASHINGTON

January 26, 1994

Greetings and congratulations to the staff, volunteers, and friends of Saint Mary of Nazareth Hospital Center as you celebrate 100 years of devoted service.

Your long-standing dedication has helped to save countless lives and give comfort to many. All who are associated with Saint Mary of Nazareth Hospital Center and its fine work have earned the respect and trust of a grateful community.

America's future well-being requires accessible and affordable health care that meets the needs of all of our people. We will need your help as we work to make health care available to everyone, control skyrocketing costs, and continue to provide the best service possible. I am pleased to commend citizens like you, who contribute everyday to improving the health of your fellow Americans.

Best wishes for great success in the years ahead.

Bill Clinton

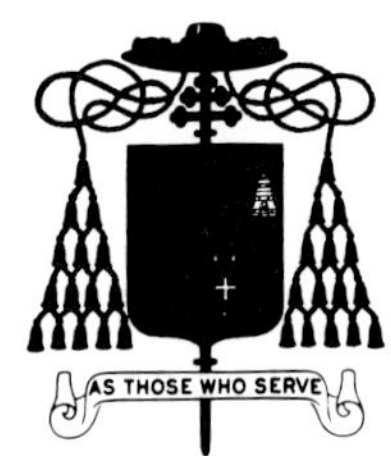

1555 North State Parkway
Chicago, Illinois 60610

January 21, 1994

Dear Friends of Saint Mary of Nazareth
Hospital Center:

On the occasion of the Centennial Anniversary of Saint Mary of Nazareth Hospital Center, it is my pleasure and privilege to extend to you my heartfelt congratulations, best wishes and promise of prayers.

The theme of the program book marking this special milestone, -- "A History of Healing, A Future of Care," -- aptly describes the commitment to providing compassionate, quality healthcare which is the hallmark of St. Mary's. The Center's dedication to these values has been a precious gift to our community over these many years.

I wish to take this opportunity to express my deep gratitude to the Sisters, medical staff, administration, employees, friends and extended family of St. Mary's for their superb support of the Catholic healthcare ministry within the Archdiocese over these many years.

Know of my friendship and support for all of you engaged in this humanitarian effort. May God be close to you, and to those you serve, today and always.

With cordial good wishes, I remain

Sincerely yours in Christ,

Joseph Card. Bernardin

Archbishop of Chicago

Centennial Anniversary
St. Mary of Nazareth Hospital Center
1894 - 1994

MESSAGES

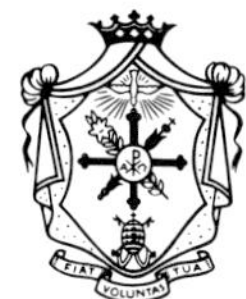

SISTERS OF THE HOLY FAMILY OF NAZARETH

353 North River Road
Des Plaines, Illinois 60016-1291

Sacred Heart Province

Dear Sisters, Staff and Friends,

Anniversaries provide us the opportunity to remember, to give thanks and to celebrate.

It was over 100 years ago that Blessed Mary of Jesus the Good Shepherd, (Frances Siedliska) arrived in Chicago to begin the work of the Sisters of the Holy Family of Nazareth in America.

Her vision of love in ministry to families was but a nineteen year old dream when on May 6, 1894 Saint Mary of Nazareth Hospital was opened. And now, 100 years later, we give thanks and celebrate everyone who has fostered and promoted the ideals and mission that have made Saint Mary's the institution of care and concern that it is today.

It seems especially fitting that the centennial of the hospital should occur during the International Year of the Family.

From birth to death, in illness and health, at every moment sacred in the life of a family, Saint Mary's has provided not only an open door, but a welcoming heart to all who have become part of their family: patients, nurses, physicians and employees. Together in love for 100 years, Saint Mary's has accepted challenges, surmounted difficulties, pioneered innovations and assumed responsibility to provide a caring family atmosphere in the healing ministry.

May all who enter the hospital in future days and generations continue to experience that same love that inspired the early pioneers of the hospital.

We pray that Saint Mary's remain a citadel of care and place of peace. More than a building, may the heart of Saint Mary's beat with compassion for families of every nation, race and creed.

"May this undertaking, begun for the glory of God,
be acceptable" now and forever.
(Words of Blessed Mary of Jesus the Good Shepherd
May 8, 1901)

Congratulations!

Sister M. Lucille
+
Sisters

ARCHDIOCESE OF CHICAGO

Episcopal Vicariate V

6101 South 75th Avenue - BOX 040
Summit-Argo, IL 60501-1628
708-458-5116
FAX 708-563-0691

Sister Stella Louise, C.S.F.N.
St. Mary of Nazareth Hospital Center
2233 West Division Street
Chicago, IL 60622

Dear Sister Stella Louise,

For over one hundred years the Sisters of the Holy Family of Nazareth have been living witnesses to the love of Christ for his sisters and brothers in need, and to the peace and joy that Christ brings to those who serve Him with love. Although their hands were already overworked by their varied apostolate of teaching youth and caring for the aged with a faith as strong as that of their holy foundress, they dared to establish Saint Mary of Nazareth Hospital in 1894 because they could not resist the constant pleas of God's children who cried, "Sister, we are sick, help us!"

May God bless you, Sisters, for your love and generosity. May you see and enjoy your reward here on earth in the daily miracles of life which you witness at Saint Mary of Nazareth Hospital Center.

The Hospital Center is not just another health institution. It is a Catholic institution, born of a love for God and neighbor, prompted and inspired not by mere humanitarian or philanthropic motives but by a desire to witness to Christ and His Church on earth.

Who is it who followed Christ? Thousands who were intrigued by the message of Christ, Blessed are the poor - the sorrowing - the humble - those who hunger and thirst for holiness - the merciful - the pure - the persecuted - the insulted.

To accept this one must have Faith, Hope and Love! Saint Mary of Nazareth Hospital Center is a citadel of Faith, Hope and Love.

Sisters, for one hundred years you along with your entire hospital staff have witnessed so nobly to Christ.

Thank you! God bless you!

Sincerely yours in Christ,

+ Alfred L. Abramowicz

Most Rev. Alfred L. Abramowicz
Auxiliary Bishop of Chicago

February 10, 1994

ARCHDIOCESE OF CHICAGO

Vicar for Regional Services
Vicar General

Post Office Box 1979
Chicago, Illinois 60690

(312) 751-8271
Fax (312) 337-6379

April, 1994

Sister Stella Louise, CSFM
President and Chief Executive Officer
Saint Mary of Nazareth Hospital Center
2233 West Division Street
Chicago, Illinois 60622-3086

Dear Sister Stella Louise:

I would like to extend to you and the Sisters of the Holy Family of Nazareth congratulations and best wishes on the 100th Anniversary of St. Mary of Nazareth Hospital Center.

The Sisters of the Holy Family of Nazareth have given their all in fulfilling their mission in healthcare to the people of Chicago over the past century. As you look forward to your next 100 years of service please know you have my support and prayers.

Sincerely yours in Christ,

Most Reverend John R. Gorman
Vicar General/Vicar for Regional Services

MESSAGES

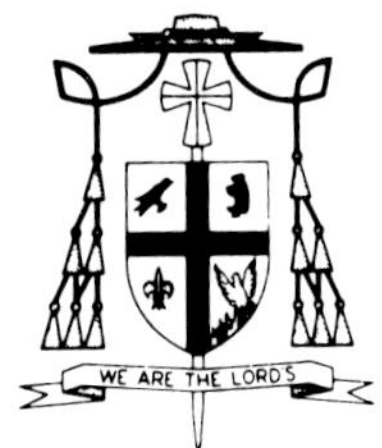

BISHOP WILTON D. GREGORY
POST OFFICE BOX 733 + SOUTH HOLLAND, IL 60473-0733 + 708/339-2474

Sunday 16 January, 1994

Sister Stella Louise, C.S.F.N.
Office of the President and Chief Executive Officer
Saint Mary of Nazareth Hospital
2233 West Division Street
Chicago, Illinois 60622-3086

Dear Sister Stella Louise,

It is my personal pleasure to send this letter of congratulations to you and to the entire Administration, Staff, and community of the Sisters of the Holy Family of Nazareth who, along with yourself, are observing the centennial of Saint Mary of Nazareth Hospital Center this calendar year of 1994.

On more than one occasion, I have witnessed, first hand, the extraordinary dedication and gentle spirit which are hallmarks of this vital institution of healing and service in the Archdiocese of Chicago. During the ten years of my ministry as Auxiliary Bishop of the Archdiocese, I was repeatedly aware of the commitment of the Sisters of the Holy Family of Nazareth in caring for the people of God in the Archdiocese through your teaching, healing, and prayerful apostolates of service. Certainly none of those ministries has a more visible impact on the lives of the people of the Archdiocese than does the great history of St. Mary of Nazareth Hospital.

I congratulate you and assure you of both my esteem and prayers during this your centennial observance.

With cordial good wishes, Sister Stella Louise, may I remain,

Yours in Christ,

+Wilton D. Gregory, S.L.D.,
Bishop-Designate of Belleville

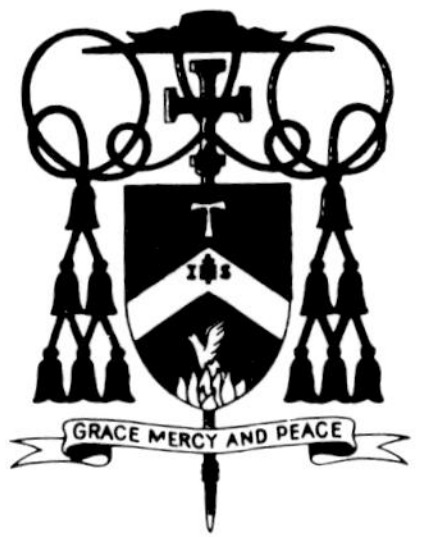

730 North Wabash Avenue
Chicago, Illinois 60611

January 13, 1994

Sister Stella Louise, CSFN
President and CEO
Saint Mary of Nazareth Hospital
2233 West Division Street
Chicago, IL 60622-3086

Dear Sister Stella Louise,

I wish to congratulate you and all of those who have worked so hard to make Saint Mary of Nazareth Hospital an outstanding center for healing for the last one hundred years. Your centennial publication, "A History of Healing, A Future of Care", says so well all that you have done and plan to do.

You have ministered to the needs of a community that has changed many times in the one hundred years and at each time you - Sisters, employees and medical staff - have made the adjustments to make your care available to all those in the community. As the world, the community, and healthcare change, once again I am sure that your good work will persevere and continue.

For all that you have done and that you will do, I extend my prayers and congratulations. May the Lord continue to bless your future care.

With every best wish, I am

Sincerely yours in Our Lord,

Most Reverend Timothy J. Lyne
Auxiliary Bishop of Chicago and
Episcopal Vicar for Vicariate II

TJL/nm

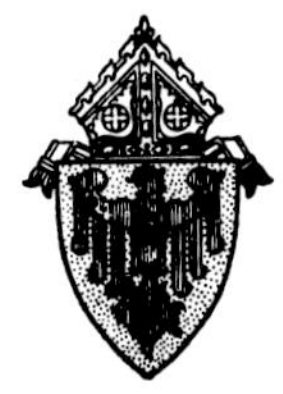

ARCHDIOCESE OF CHICAGO

Office of the Episcopal Vicar
1048 North Campbell Avenue
Chicago, Illinois 60622
(312) 486-6966

February 1, 1994

Sr. Stella Louise, C.S.F.N.
St. Mary of Nazareth Hospital
2233 W. Division St.
Chicago, Illinois 60622

Dear Sr. Stella Louise, C.S.F.N.,

St. Mary of Nazareth Hospital Center is celebrating a century (1894-1994) of healing, and it is your Congregation of Sisters who have made this century of healing ministry even more significant to all of us.

This souvenir centennial publication "A History of Healing, A Future of Care" is a testimony of the Gospel we preach translated into action in our Society. As Jesus went about casting out demons and healing the sick as a sign that the Kingdom of God was at hand, so the ministry of the Sisters of the Holy Family of Nazareth for the last 100 years has been a sign of your public ministry, an expression of your vowed life to bring about the Kingdom of God. Your history of healing is a beautiful history.

I am honored to include my sincere greetings and congratulations on this important milestone in your ministry. I have been privileged to serve as a member of the Governing Board for several years and I have been impressed with the spirit and dedication after the example of your Foundress, Blessed Frances Siedliska, C.S.F.N.

May the Lord, the Good Shepherd, continue to bless and guide St. Mary of Nazareth Hospital Center in its next century of ministry of healing.

Sincerely yours in Christ,

+Plácido Rodríguez, cmf.

Most Rev. Plácido Rodríguez, C.M.F.
Auxiliary Bishop of Chicago

PR:gpp

PAUL SIMON
ILLINOIS

COMMITTEES:
LABOR AND HUMAN RESOURCES
JUDICIARY
FOREIGN RELATIONS
BUDGET
INDIAN AFFAIRS

United States Senate
WASHINGTON, DC 20510-1302

February 3, 1994

Saint Mary of Nazareth Hospital Center
2233 West Division Street
Chicago, Illinois 60622-3086

Dear Friends:

It gives me great pleasure to add my congratulations to the many who will send you greetings on your 100th anniversary.

Saint Mary of Nazareth Hospital Center has been a place of true healing in the communities of the near northwest side of Chicago. Its strength and range of services has grown remarkably over the years, and it has been steadfast in its mission to minister to those most in need.

There are those who say health care reform will be one of the ultimate tests of the morality of our government. As we grapple with this great test, we will do well to be guided by the moral compass of the hundreds of dedicated souls who have served through the years at Saint Mary of Nazareth.

I hope that our city will continue to find comfort in Saint Mary's humane care -- while we have far less need for its charity -- for many years into the future.

My thanks and best wishes.

Cordially,

Paul Simon
U. S. Senator

PS/jlw

462 Dirksen Building
Washington, DC 20510-1302
202/224-2152
TDD: 202/224-5469

230 S. Dearborn
Kluczynski Bldg., 38th Floor
Chicago, IL 60604
312/353-4952
TDD: 312/786-0308

3 West Old Capitol Plaza
Suite 1
Springfield, IL 62701
217/492-4960
TDD: 217/544-7524

250 West Cherry
Room 115-B
Carbondale, IL 62901
618/457-3653

LUIS V. GUTIERREZ
4TH DISTRICT, ILLINOIS
COMMITTEE ON BANKING, FINANCE AND URBAN AFFAIRS
SUBCOMMITTEES:
HOUSING AND COMMUNITY DEVELOPMENT
CONSUMER CREDIT AND INSURANCE
COMMITTEE ON VETERANS' AFFAIRS
SUBCOMMITTEES:
HOSPITALS AND HEALTH CARE
OVERSIGHT AND INVESTIGATIONS

Congress of the United States
House of Representatives
Washington, DC 20515-1304

1208 LONGWORTH BUILDING
WASHINGTON, DC 20515
(202) 225-8203
3181 NORTH ELSTON AVE.
CHICAGO, IL 60618
(312) 509-0999

February 28, 1994

Sister Stella Louise, CSFN
President and Chief Executive Officer
Saint Mary of Nazareth Hospital Center
2233 W. Division Street
Chicago, Illinois 60622-3086

Dear Sister Stella:

I am honored to have this opportunity to congratulate you and the Sisters of the HOly Family of Nazareth on your century of serving the community and ministering to the healthcare needs of the people of Chicago.

I have been pleased to work with you and your staff during my tenure as Alderman of the 26th Ward and now as Congressman of the 4th Congressional District.

With healthcare on the top of our nation's agenda, I look forward to continuing to work with Saint Mary of Nazareth Hospital to evaluate and implement a national healthcare system.

Congratulations once again.

Sincerely,

Luis V. Gutierrez
Member of Congress

LVG:lb

DAN ROSTENKOWSKI
5TH DISTRICT, ILLINOIS

COMMITTEES:
CHAIRMAN
COMMITTEE ON
WAYS AND MEANS

CHAIRMAN
JOINT COMMITTEE ON
TAXATION

Congress of the United States
House of Representatives
Washington, DC 20515-1305

January 26, 1994

Sister Stella Louise, CSFN
President and Chief Executive Officer
St. Mary's of Nazareth Hospital
2233 West Division Street
Chicago, Illinois 60622-3086

Dear Sister Stella Louise:

Thank you for the chance to publicly congratulate St. Mary's of Nazareth Hospital on its centennial anniversary. St. Mary's has a special spot in my heart. I was born there, and although I have no recollection of my stay, reliable sources tell me that I made more than my share of noise in the nursery.

Reliable sources also tell me that I received the very best of care. This comes as no surprise. St. Mary's and the Sisters of the Holy Family of Nazareth have been providing top quality medical treatment ever since that day one hundred years ago when the hospital first opened its doors.

What distinguishes St. Mary's is not simply the technical sophistication of the doctors and nurses who work there. Just as important -- maybe even more important -- is the fact that at St. Mary's patients not only receive health care, they are cared for, as well. This is an aspect of modern medicine which has, unfortunately, been grossly neglected. The clinical and financial side of health care have overwhelmed the emotional side. Too many in the health care profession have forgotten that medicine is, in the final analysis, as much about kindness and compassion as it is about knowledge and technology.

You've never lost sight of this at St. Mary's. For a hundred years, the people of Chicago have had the inestimable security of knowing that in time of sickness St. Mary's will always be there. I congratulate you on your success. But, above all else, I thank you.

Sincerely yours,

Dan Rostenkowski
Member of Congress

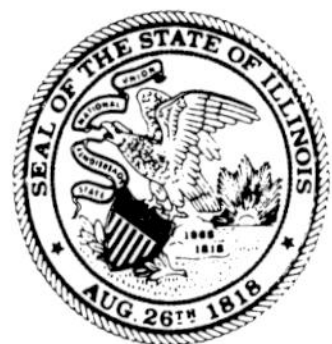

STATE OF ILLINOIS

OFFICE OF THE GOVERNOR

SPRINGFIELD 62706

JIM EDGAR
GOVERNOR

April 1994

Greetings:

As Governor of the State of Illinois, it is my pleasure to join the Sisters of the Holy Family of Nazareth in celebrating Saint Mary of Nazareth Hospital Center's 100th anniversary.

The hospital provides a vital healthcare ministry to the people of Chicago. Over the past century, the Saint Mary of Nazareth Hospital has served with a dedication that pays tribute to your faith in God. I applaud your vision and flexibility as you respond to the changing healthcare market.

On behalf of the citizens of Illinois, please accept my best wishes for an enjoyable celebration and another fruitful year of service.

Best regards,

Jim Edgar

Jim Edgar
GOVERNOR

Printed on Recycled Paper

CHAPTER I

Szpital Polski

Abundant work in the city's new mills, factories, tanneries and packing houses drew Polish immigrants by the hundreds of thousands across the Atlantic to the Midwest and to the booming, bustling Chicago of the late 1800s.

They were together in a new land, with fresh opportunities. Chicago's Polish families of 1890 had much of what they had sought when they left Poland: spiritual guidance in Catholic parishes, jobs, social and political freedom, housing they could afford, some schooling, ample food. They worked hard, and they played hard.

Clustered Polish tenements nestled near the intersection of Ashland and Chicago Avenues on the near northwest side. The edge of the city dropped away to farmland just a short distance to the west.

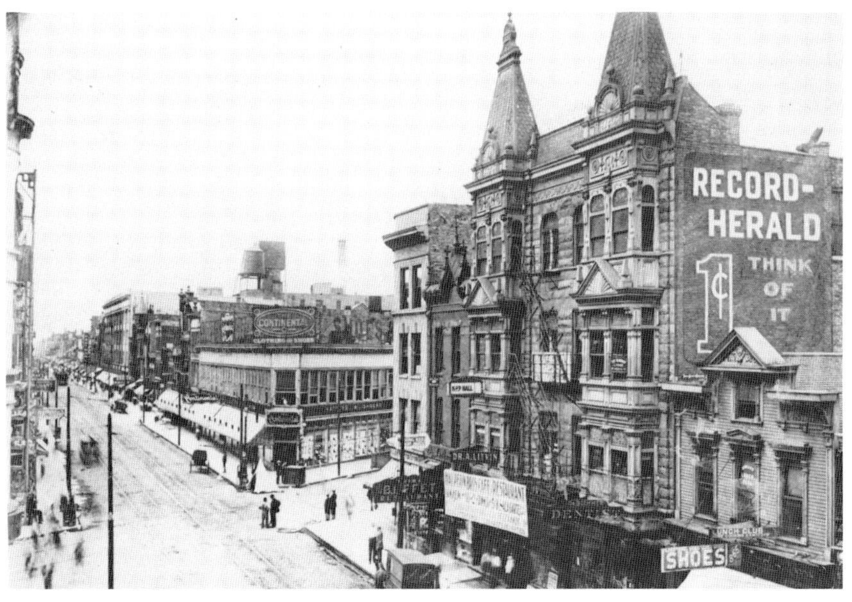

Polish immigrant neighborhood, Milwaukee and Ashland Avenues, 1911 (photo courtesy of the Chicago Historical Society)

Polish families were neighbored by Swedish, Norwegian, Slovak, German, Russian, Bohemian, Ukrainian and Jewish immigrants, and each nationality kept to themselves.

Streets were unpaved; sidewalks were of wood and tar. The well-to-do rode horseback or in carriages. Toilets were semi-public, intended mostly for nearby families. Poor sanitation bred tuberculosis, typhoid and cholera.

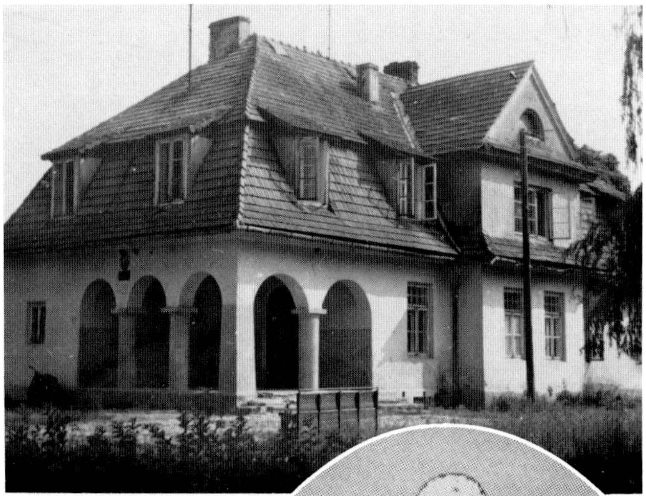

Roszkowa Wola, the Siedliska family home in Zdzary, Poland

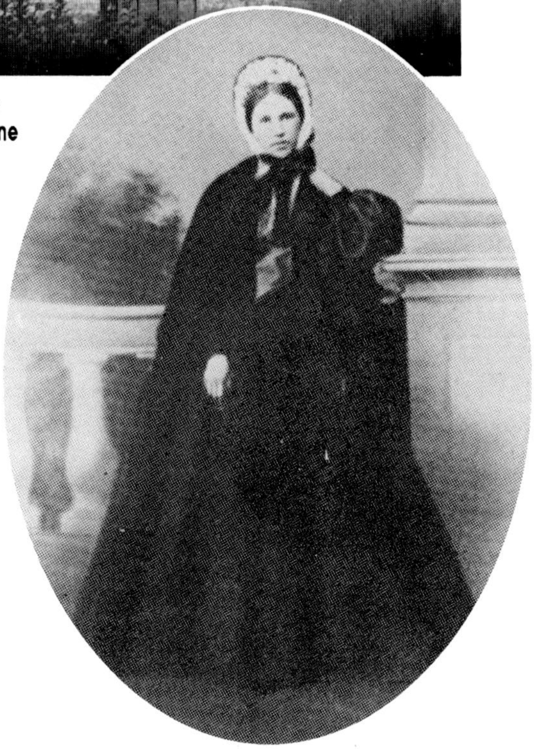

Frances Siedliska, circa 1867

Chicago needs a Polish hospital

For Polish immigrants in need of healthcare, this scrambling, prospering city of the late 19th century was not a place to seek healing. Being sick and Polish was often a lonely, distressing experience. It was nearly impossible to find medical help from people who spoke Polish. And no hospital in all of Chicago understood the Polish-Catholic culture.

As late as 1893, there were a handful of Polish doctors—but no Polish hospital and no Polish nurses.

The beginning of the solution was forged by a noblewoman born on November 12, 1842. Frances Anne Josephine Siedliska had been welcomed into the splendor and luxury of Roszkowa Wola, the family manor in central Poland.

The nation was in chaos. A Pole could not point to a map and categorically claim the territory as his country. Foreigners ruled. Just 12 years before her birth, Frances' parents lived through the tragic and ill-fated November Insurrection of 1830. Through these troubled times, Frances' father, Adolph Siedliska, a powerful tycoon, sustained his staunch Polish patriotism, siding with attempts to overthrow foreign government. Frances' mother, Cecilia Morawska, came from old aristocratic lineage.

Many highborn Poles had fled to France and returned to Poland, having absorbed the anti-ecclesiastical philosophies of Voltaire and Rousseau. Adolph and Cecilia Siedliska had also succumbed to this thinking.

Frances turns to God

Her future among the socially elite was being planned by her parents, but Frances glimpsed another life. While growing up in such material splendor—her parents' palatial estate and a life of wealth, culture and private governesses—the frail and pensive Frances chose a different path.

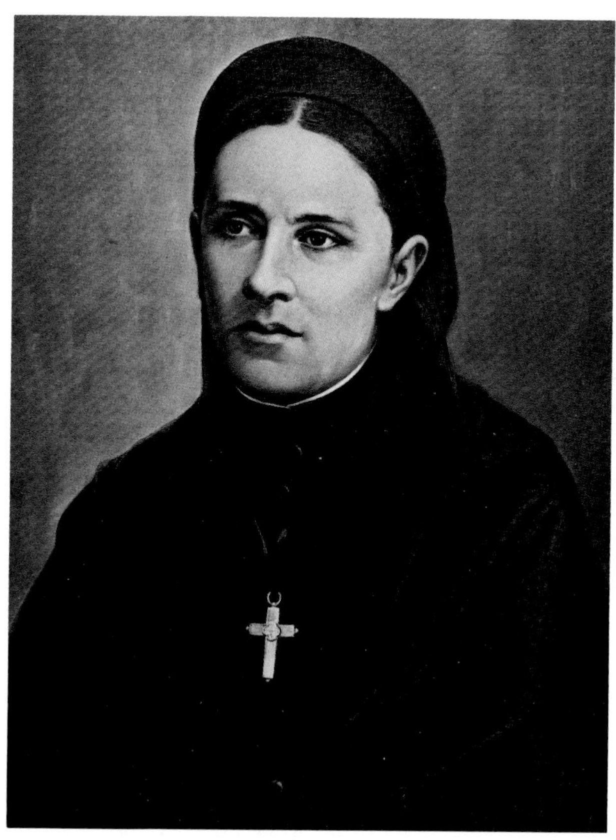

Blessed Mary of Jesus the Good Shepherd (Frances Siedliska), Foundress of the Congregation of Sisters of the Holy Family of Nazareth (shown in the Congregation's first habit)

She became devoted to her Church and to her country, and struggled against the wishes of her family. God came into her life through the influence of an intense Capuchin, Father Leander Lendzian, who

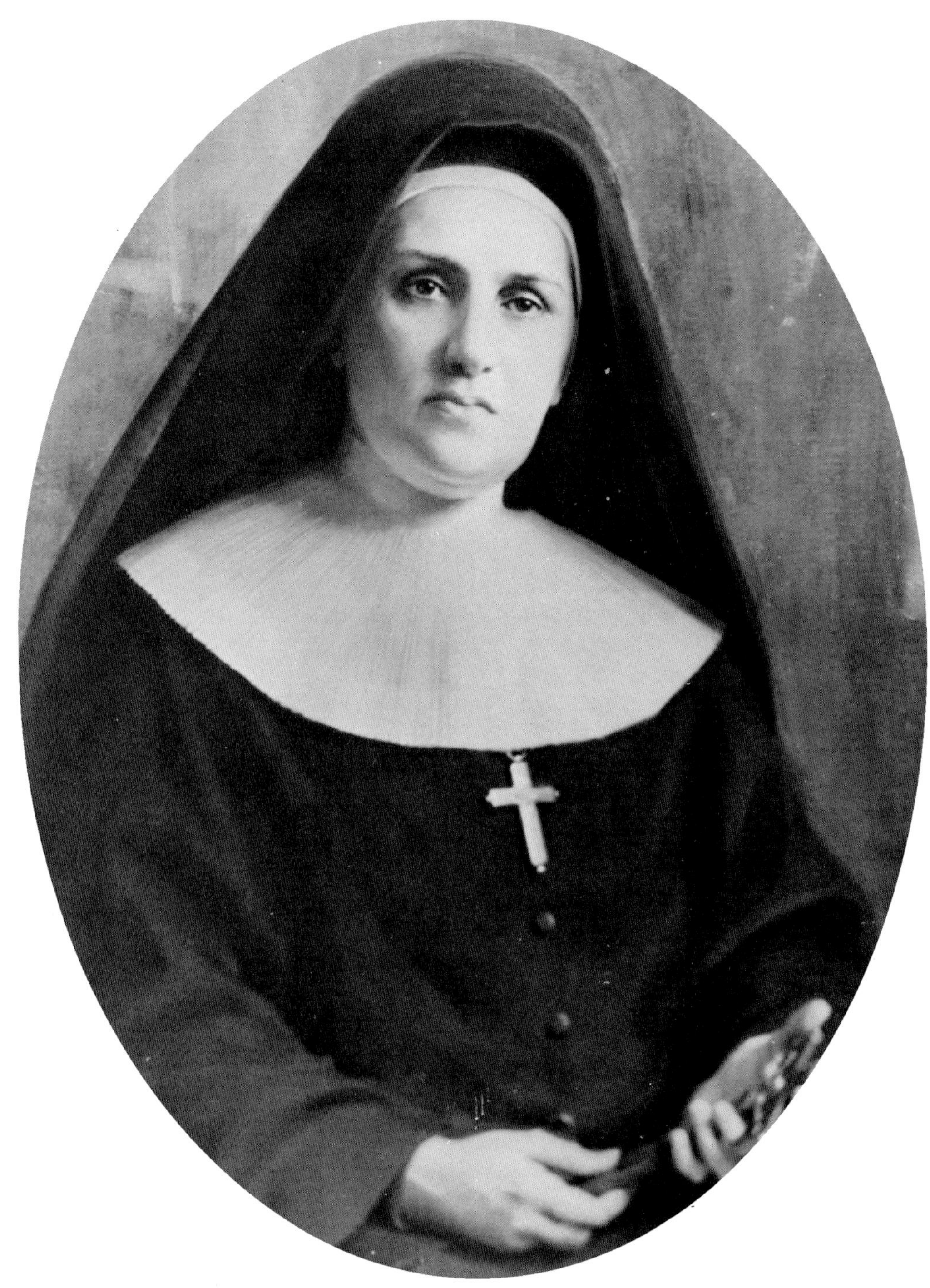

When the Sisters came to America, a bishop suggested they wear a more elaborate habit and cover their hair, to distinguish them from widows. The Mother Foundress is shown wearing the revised habit, worn by the Sisters until the 1960s.

prepared her for her first Holy Communion. A desire to serve God in the religious life was awakened in her. Worldly temptations, criticism and derision failed to dissuade her.

After her father died, Frances consecrated herself to God's service and took the name Mary Frances. In Rome in 1875, when she was 33, Pope Pius IX allowed her to establish a new order called the Institute of Mary of Nazareth, later to be known as the Congregation of Sisters of the Holy Family of Nazareth. Mother Mary Frances and four pioneer followers modeled their lives on the quiet life and virtues of the Holy Family. Guided by Father Anthony Lechert, the Sisters taught religion to children, instructed converts, and conducted retreats for women.

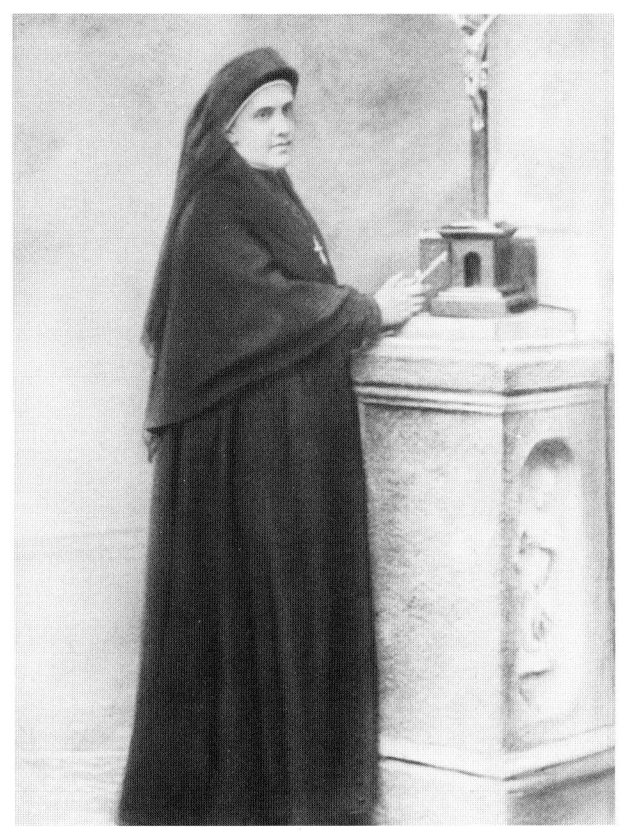

Mother Foundress, 1889

On April 19, 1880, Mother Frances submitted "A Brief Plan of the Institute of Mary of Nazareth," the first official presentation to the Church of the project of her Congregation. Care of the sick in a hospital setting was not one of the works of mercy she outlined. At a time when many felt that the Church was being oppressed, the Papacy insulted, and contempt for God and impiety were causing division, her proposal aimed to lead souls to the knowledge and love of the church of Jesus Christ.

As new candidates entered the

A Homecoming...and History Comes Alive

Mother Foundress was often depicted with an African-American child under her cape. Little concrete information was known, although a sculpture of the Foundress and 'her little adopted daughter Grace' was unveiled in 1993 at Mother Frances Hospital in Tyler, Texas. So you can imagine the surprise of the Public Relations Staff on receiving an intriguing call in early 1994 from a woman seeking information about her mother and aunt, Yolande and Grace Charleston, young African-American orphans raised in Poland around the turn of the century by the Sisters of the Holy Family of Nazareth!

On February 17,1994, Sisters from Saint Mary's, Provincial Superior Sister Lucille, historian Sister Edith, archivist Sister Gemma and other Sisters from the provincialate in Des Plaines gathered at the hospital to meet Lauretta Frances Travis and Gloria Wilson, Yolande's daughters. The women are nieces of Grace Charleston, the child thought to be depicted. Also in attendance was Lauretta's son Albert, whose interest in his grandmother's past prompted Mrs. Travis' phone call to Saint Mary's.

The Charleston sisters were born in New York City, and then brought to Poland and adopted by Mother Foundress. Grace remained in Europe and became a Sister of the Congregation, but Yolande returned to the U.S. in 1910. Still under the legal guardianship of the sisters, she initially attended Saint Mary's school of nursing. After one year, she received Mother Lauretta's permission to transfer to Provident Hospital's school, where there would be other African-Americans. She graduated in 1914 and worked through the years as a nurse, social worker, probation officer and court interpreter for the federal court.

Continued on page 30

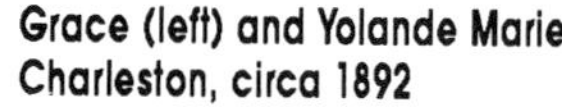

Grace (left) and Yolande Marie Charleston, circa 1892

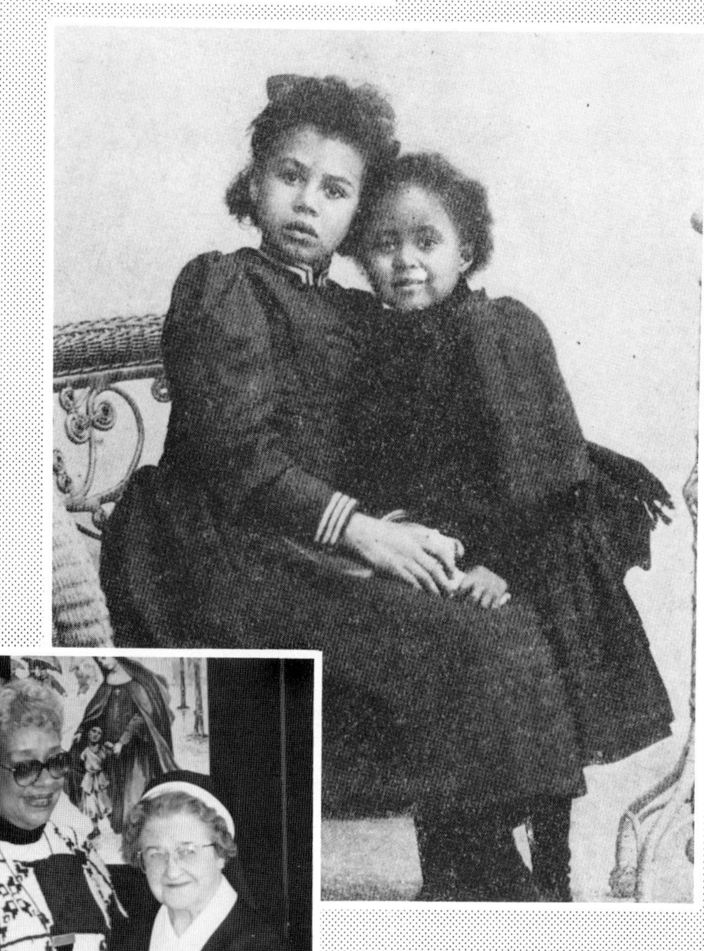

Sister Agnes renews her acquaintance with Lauretta Travis. She remembered meeting her and her mother in the late 1930's. In the background is an illustration of Mother Foundress with Grace.

A Homecoming continued

She could speak Polish, French and Italian. She married Thomas Wilson, a writer for the *Chicago Defender,* in 1917. Sister Amata Menge is listed as a witness on her marriage certificate. Lauretta Frances is named after Mother Foundress and Mother Lauretta.

Yolande's roots always remained with Saint Mary's, and her daughters have wonderful childhood memories of coming here to visit their mother's 'family.' Gloria Wilson said, 'We used to go to Saint Mary's like others went to grandmother's house–for Thanksgiving, Christmas, Easter... The Sisters were the only family we knew. We'd take the street car from Morgan Park. Were we spoiled! The Sisters would travel to see us make our First Communion, Confirmation, and for special occasions.' It seemed appropriate that Sister Sandra Marie greeted them, 'Hello, cousins!'

Of special interest to the Sisters was trying to match the Wilson sisters' information about their aunt with congregational archives. They all excitedly poured over old photos, postcards and documents.

Gloria Wilson said, 'This has certainly stirred up many emotions for me, and answered pieces of the puzzle I have wondered about over the years.' Lauretta Travis echoed her words, 'Yesterday was an absolutely one-of-a-kind day. I never stopped feeling like visiting royalty. Albert was really awed and could not stop looking at the (display). I believe yesterday was the very first time he could relate to the stories he had heard all of his life.'

One simple phone call has led to international interest, as congregational historians in France, Poland and Italy—in addition to Des Plaines—have begun searching through old records to help get an accurate historical recounting. It seems exceptionally fitting to have discovered this link to our past during our centennial year and the International Year of the Family.

order, Mother Frances worked unceasingly. In 1881 she opened a convent in Krakow. By 1885 her apostolic energy brought her to the United States for the first of three journeys. Not only were she and her 11 Sisters leaving behind the security of their beloved homeland, but when they crossed the Atlantic and came to Chicago they were entering mission territory.

Mother Frances comes to the heart of America

Ten years after the order's founding and immediately upon reaching Chicago, the Congregation established St. Josephat's School and Orphanage. Word of their good work spread quickly. Several local parishes and distant bishops requested Mother Frances to develop more schools. Always proceeding efficiently, she took to every new project with a keen interest. Eventually, there would be 28 Chicago schools staffed by Sisters of the Holy Family of Nazareth.

Most of the children taught and cared for were from immigrant families. When family members were ill or injured, they often turned to the Sisters who shared simple home remedies and made visits to the bedridden.

Chicago's hospitals were strained and inadequate at best. They were often closed to various immigrant groups. The Sisters regularly visited ailing Polish immigrants in the local hospitals that did accept them. They were accompanied by Mother Mary Lauretta Lubowicka, the newly appointed 27-year-old Provincial for the United States. In addition to their native tongue, most of the Sisters could also speak French and Italian. Some of them could speak German. Thus they were quite helpful, interpreting the doctor's diagnoses and recommendations. Still, Polish immigrants needed a hospital where they could feel at home with their own people and where they could communicate their needs to the physician in their native language.

When Mother Frances made her second trip to the United States in 1889, she became very much aware of the need for a hospital for immigrants. Chicago's bishop,

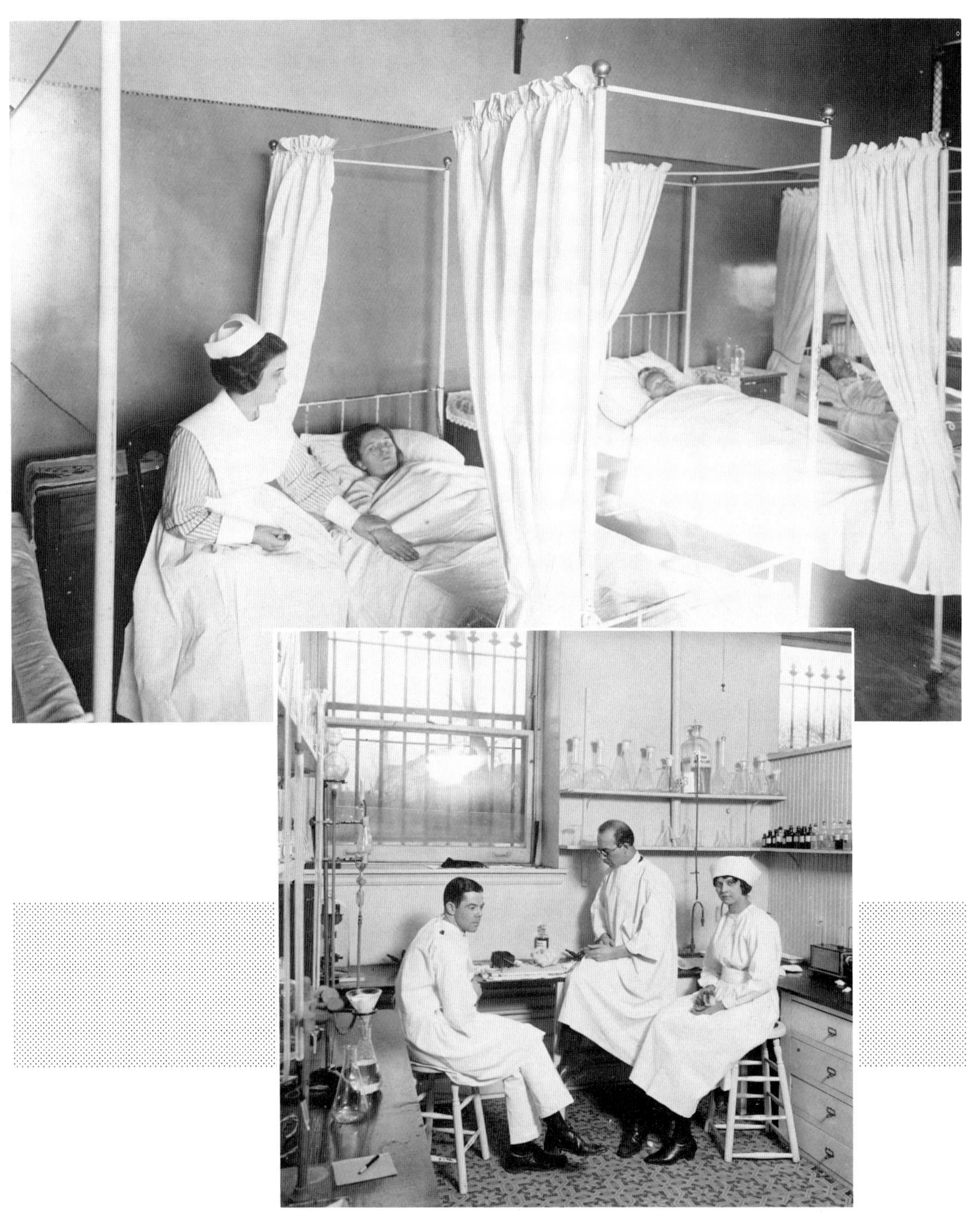

the Most Reverend Patrick J. Feehan, DD, appealed to her. Envisioning another branch on the tree of apostolic works, Mother Frances told her Sisters that the will of God was leading them to accept a new ministry in addition to that of teaching children and young women. This new apostolate would be devoted to care of the sick in a proper hospital setting, in familiar religious and cultural surroundings.

The pragmatic Mother Frances also strongly suggested to the Sisters that they learn to speak English in order to facilitate their work and to receive American citizenship, as she had done.

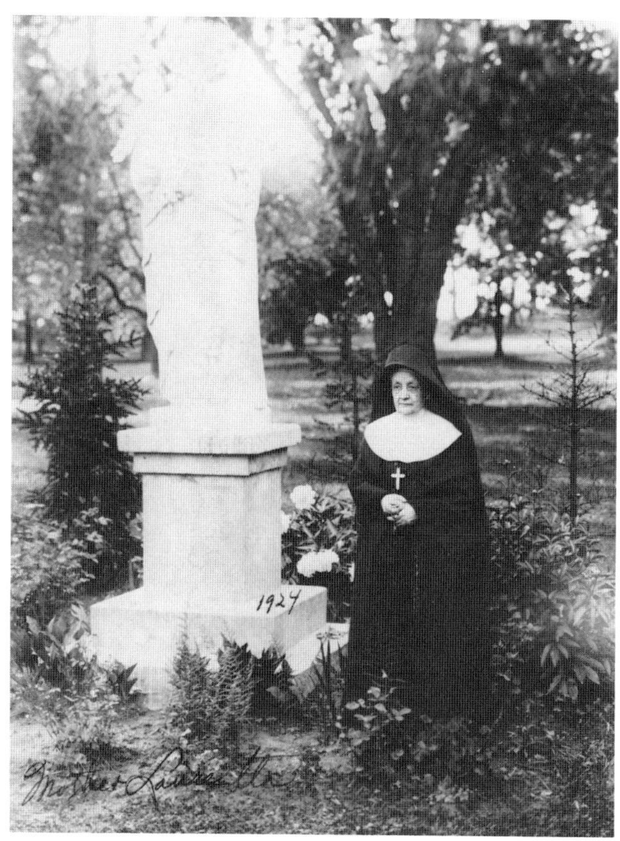

Mother Mary Lauretta Lubowicka, successor to Mother Frances as Superior General of the Congregation, 1924

Mother Lauretta to supervise

By the late summer of 1890, Mother Frances had entrusted the task of starting a hospital to Mother Lauretta. It was to be a fortuitous collaboration. Mother Lauretta entered wholeheartedly into the Foundress' thinking. She had the same intuitions, the same concerns, and similar solutions to vexing problems. Throughout her 80 years, Mother Lauretta would demonstrate an ability to cut through incidentals, identify the important issues of any situation, and get to the heart of the matter. Twenty years younger than Mother Frances, this diminutive Sister (less than five feet tall), with her penetrating eyes and

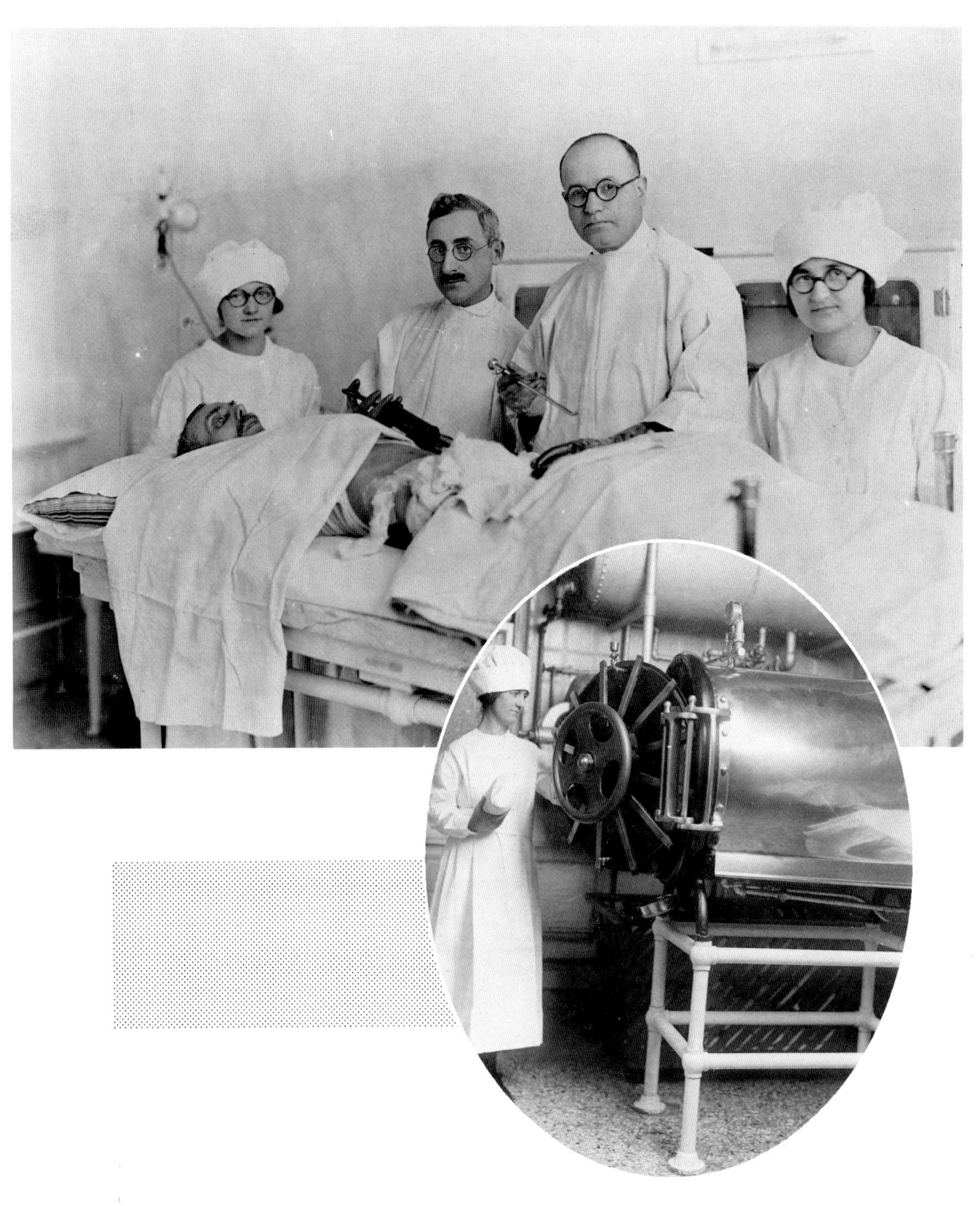

indomitable will, ably set about realizing the vision of the Foundress.

With the help of Mother Mary Paula and Mother Mary Columba, Mother Lauretta began the daunting task of starting the new hospital by overcoming such obstacles as incorporation of the Congregation under the laws of the State of Illinois on January 5, 1892.

Then came the difficult task of raising funds for a building. Despite unsettled economic conditions, the Polish and other citizens of Chicago responded to the call. By August 1892, the Sisters had been given the deed to the property at what is now 1714-22 West Division Street.

The location was far from ideal; the elevated train was also there. Earsplitting noise was anything but conducive to convalescence. The three-story brick house was abandoned and badly in need of repair. Formerly for residences, the structure was slowly put into shape as a 24-bed hospital. It included a reception area, dispensary, laundry, kitchen, chapel, operating room, bathrooms and doctors' offices.

Early in 1894, the doctors who wanted to open the hospital informally met several times to discuss the facility. Less than a month before the hospital was opened, the first official doctors' conference was held to establish principles of the new institution. The physicians were aware of Mother Lauretta's emphasis on the hospital's universal character; it was to accept patients of all religions, races and nationalities. At this meeting, the doctors pledged their services free of charge for one year so that patients of little or no means could be treated.

Five days before opening, the hospital was officially given its name, and the first governing board, chief of the medical staff (Dr. Charles G. Davis) and hospital superintendent (Mother Paula) were appointed.

Dedication day

10:00 a.m., Sunday, May 6, 1894: Bishop Patrick Feehan—who would later become the first archbishop of Chicago—dedicated Holy Family of Nazareth Hospital and offered a Mass of thanksgiving. Convent annals declare the day was beautiful and the sun shone brightly. It was a day of "city-wide

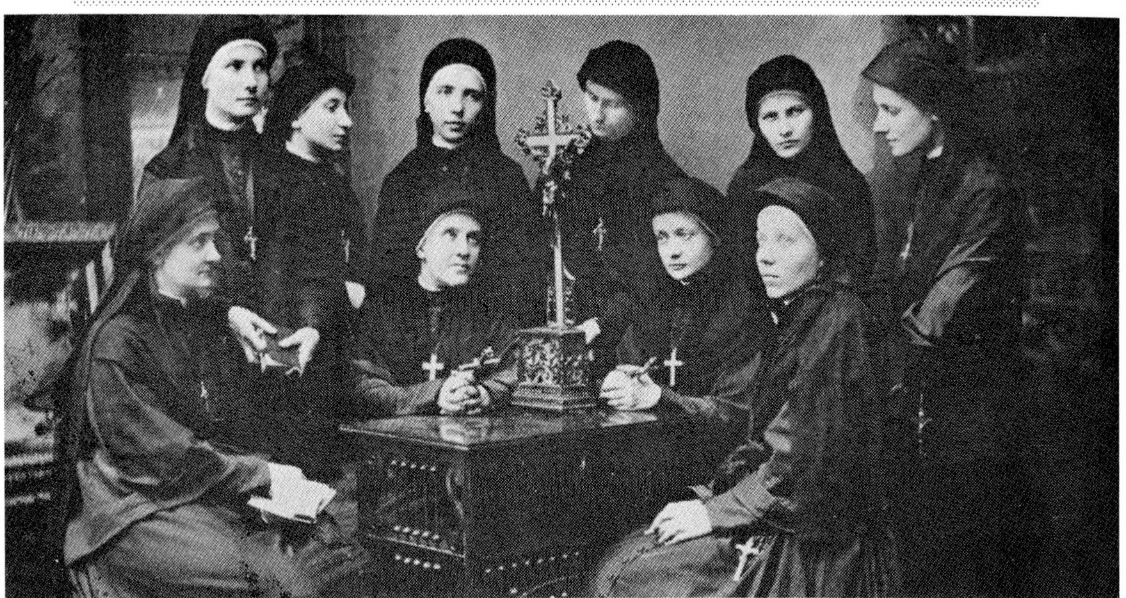

Sisters at a meeting in Chicago, 1889 (standing, left to right: Sister Bronislawa, Sister Leontyna, Mother Sofia, Sister Alberta, Mother Franciszska and Mother Teresa; seated, left to right: Mother Paula, Mother Zalozycielka, Mother Lauretta and Mother Columba) Mother Paula was the first hospital administrator and Mother Sophia the third. Sisters Lauretta, Columba and Sophia were the first three chairpersons of the governing board.

Men's ward at the first hospital with Dr. W. A. Kuflewski, Assistant Surgeon, in background

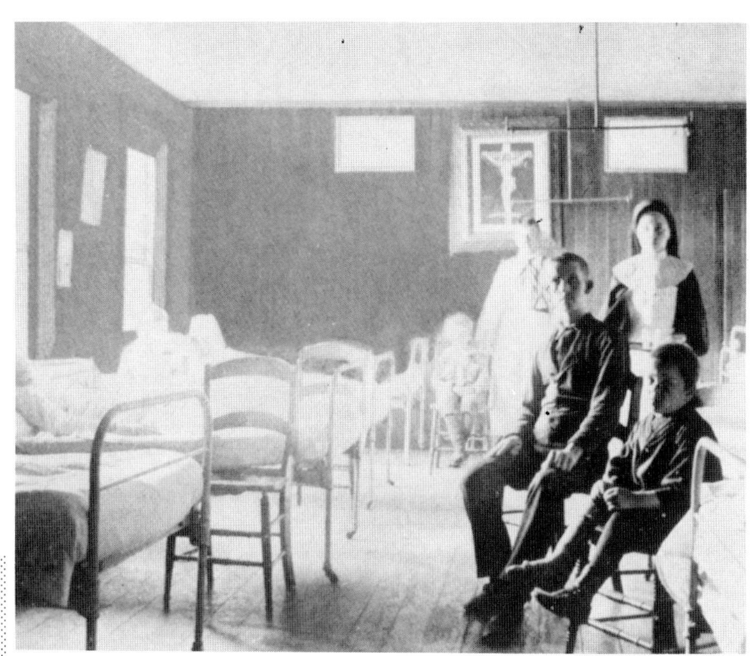

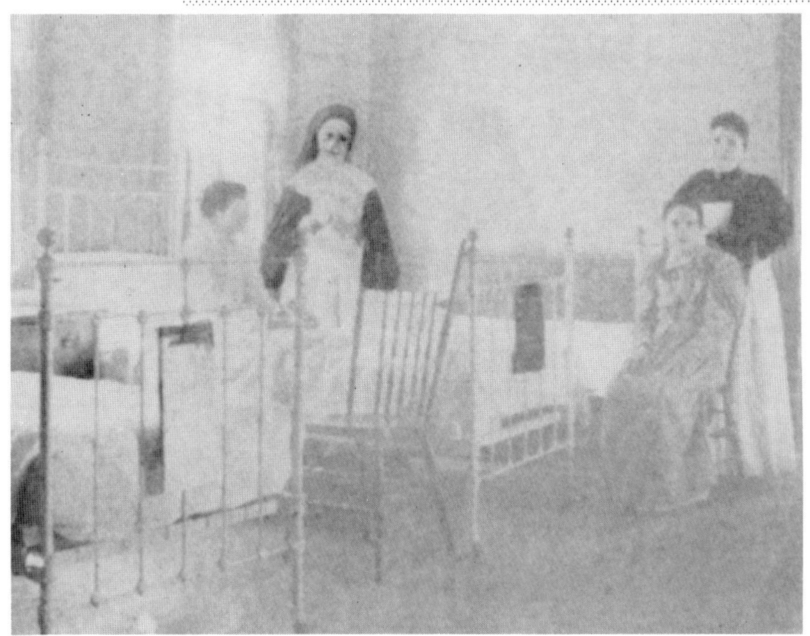

Women's ward at the first hospital with Sister Mary Cyrilla, an attending nurse, and volunteer nurse's aide

exultation" because the 24-bed hospital would alleviate a severely felt need.

Prominent civic leader and City Treasurer Peter Kiolbasa directed a large group of Chicagoans who solemnly participated in the dedicatory ceremonies.

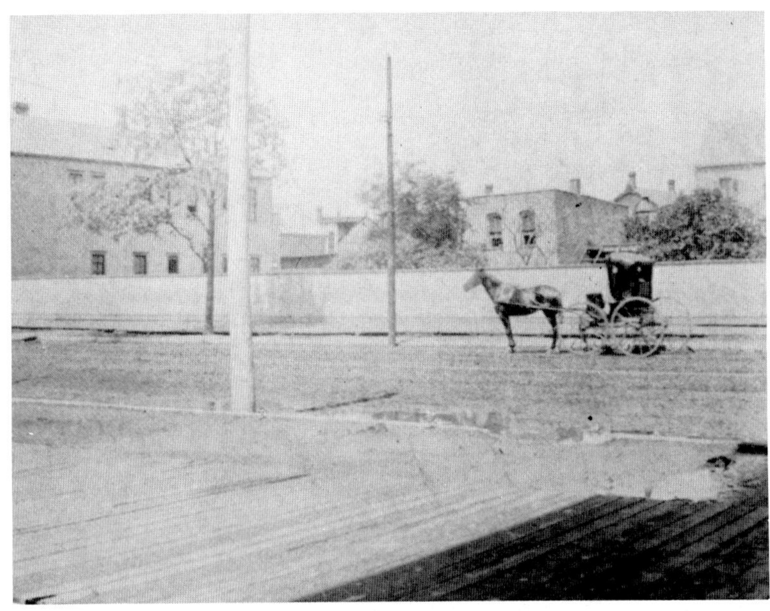
Immediate surroundings of the first hospital on Division Street—the building at the extreme left, acquired in 1899, provided rooms exclusively for women.

The German newspaper, *Englishe Illinois Staats-Zeitung,* described the hospital: "A solidly built . . . house with the unpretentious sign upon its door: '**Szpital Polski.**'"

Promptly after dedication, the hospital cared for its first patient. The register read (in Polish): "May 6, 1894—Stanley Bober, age 6, of Saint Stanislaus Kostka parish. Fractured arm, injuries of the head."

Receipts for that first day, which included care of two other patients, came to 26 cents.

The first surgery and use of anesthetic was on May 8, two days later.

None of the original Sisters was a registered nurse, and none had received special training or preparation for any of the tasks they had to perform. There were no funds for hired help, so the Sisters divided their time between bedside nursing and laundry, kitchen, and other housekeeping duties. The young postulants' main duty was to keep the entire hospital spotlessly clean. It was routine for a Sister at work in the laundry to be called to put on her apron, go upstairs to attend the sick, then immediately return to the laundry. And they worked 20- to 24-hour shifts.

The Sisters put newly admitted, acutely ill patients in an ordinary chair and carried them up three flights of stairs to the ward or to one of the five sickrooms on the second floor. Doctors carried patients to and from the operating room.

Food was in chronically short supply. Patients were sure to receive the best, while the Sisters received leftovers—when there were any. Initially, food was prepared at Holy Family Academy, four blocks away, then carried to the hospital and reheated.

The Sisters took meals whenever and wherever time and duties permitted. Only one or two Sisters enjoyed the comforts of a bed. The others rolled out mattresses or blankets, using any available place to sleep, even in the boiler room. A house was eventually donated to the Sisters; but living there proved to be an adventure, with a leaking roof and invasions of pests.

On December 31, 1894—eight months into its existence—Holy Family of Nazareth Hospital reported a total income of $126. Forty-six patients had been treated. Seventeen bills had been paid. The Sisters were forced to beg for food. Making tours with a horse-drawn buggy, they collected it themselves at least three times a week. They stood at factory entrances on paydays, asking for charity for their patients, hoping to receive a few coins.

Another building added

On her third visit to Chicago in 1896-97, Mother Frances observed that, judging by the number of patients, the hospital was becoming a fruitful branch on Nazareth's tree of apostolic ministries. Until a larger, more modern hospital could be built, an adjacent two-story frame building would expand the facilities by 20 beds, enabling the Sisters to accommodate 44 patients. Men would remain in the original hospital, while women and children would be placed in the newer one.

Their objective was not realized until 1899, when the building was finally acquired; but Mother Frances gave Mother Lauretta and Superintendent Mother Mary Sophia permission to purchase the adjacent structure.

The drawback to the acquisition was that the doctors now had to walk long distances on their rounds—between two facilities separated by a four-lot garden. As community health needs continued to grow, even the additional facilities would prove to be inadequate.

Mother Lauretta and Mother Frances had foreseen the growth and expansion of the hospital and the necessity of purchasing at least 50 lots on which to build a large, well-equipped, modern institution. And they agreed that it should remain under the patronage of the Holy Family of Nazareth.

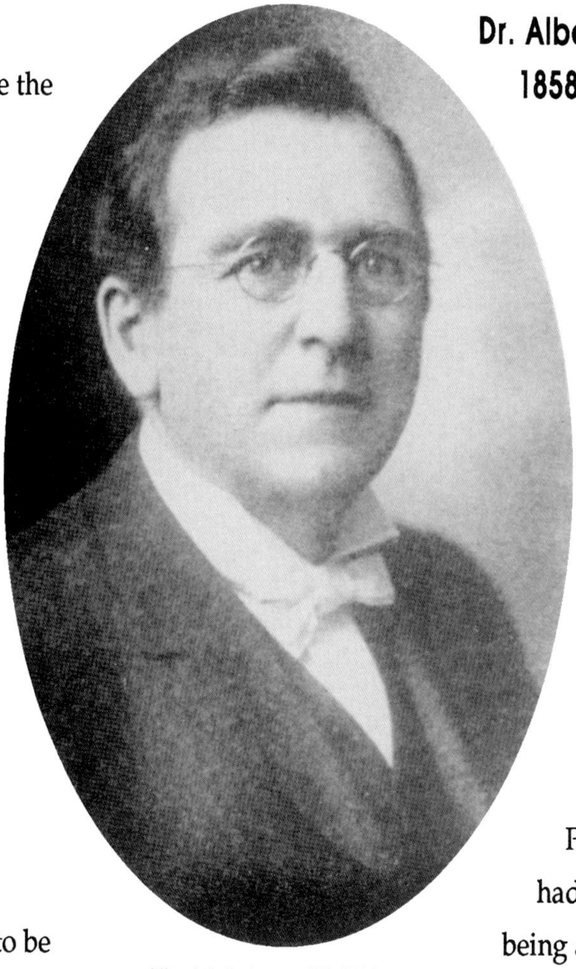

Albert J. Ochsner, MD 1858-1925

Dr. Albert J. Ochsner 1858-1925

Dr. Ochsner played an important part in the founding of the hospital. His knowledge, medical skill and experience were undoubtedly among the reasons for the substantial increase of patients at the hospital.

Physician, surgeon (he had the reputation of being a "master in the operating arena"), inventor ("Ochsner forceps"), educator and medical artist, he served as an exemplary chief of staff for 31 years. He was central to the establishment of a hospital School of Nursing.

From 1900 until his death, he occupied the position of professor of clinical surgery in the medical department of the University of Illinois. In 1900 he was elected chairman of the Section on Surgery of the American Medical Association. He subsequently held presidencies at the Clinical Congress of Surgeons of North America and the American Surgical Association.

Dr. Ochsner died July 25, 1925. His role in founding the hospital and his dedication to the highest possible professional standards made him a star of the hospital's early history.

The Women's Auxiliary

During Mother Frances' third and final visit to America, she initiated a fundraising campaign and encouraged Mother Lauretta to solicit financial help from people interested in Polish projects that would benefit their fellow countrymen. Mother Frances recommended that Mother Lauretta secure the services of professional musicians and vocalists. She indicated that recognizable talent and genuine quality in these benefit activities would draw individuals capable of making a monetary contribution.

According to Father Antonio Ricciardi, in his biography of Mother Frances: "Mother Lauretta was full of zeal and began to work energetically on these fundraising activities. Generous and magnanimous individuals in positions of leadership came to her help with financial contributions. The public support they gave encouraged others to cooperate financially. Baron E. Jerzmanowski, John and Edward De Reszke, and Countess Lubienska were in the forefront, and others followed their example by giving monetary contributions or by participating in organizing projects for this purpose." The American poet (Alfred) Joyce Kilmer (1886-1918) was an early benefactor of the hospital.

Just 10 years after the hospital opened its doors, the Women's Auxiliary was organized on November 16, 1904. Their stated purpose: "To aid the hospital in every possible way." In their pre-organization meeting, they formed a pact "to carry through the idea of charitable activity which would provide for hospital incidentals for the needy." In the beginning, members were mostly physicians' wives.

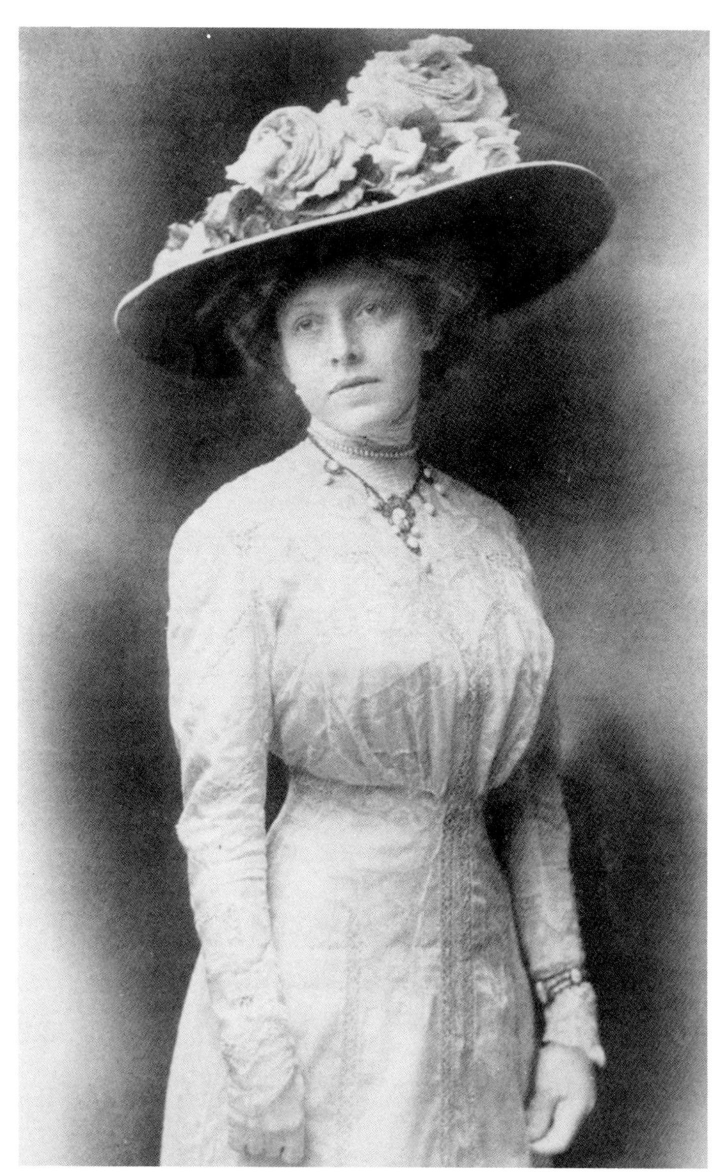

Mrs. George Mueller

The first proceeds came from a fair. It had been well publicized in Polish papers. The admission fee was ten cents, and the fee for the entire evening of "promised enjoyment" was 75 cents.

Within the first five years of its existence, the Women's Auxiliary launched an elaborate social program to acquaint illustrious patrons with the possibility of sharing the work of the hospital.

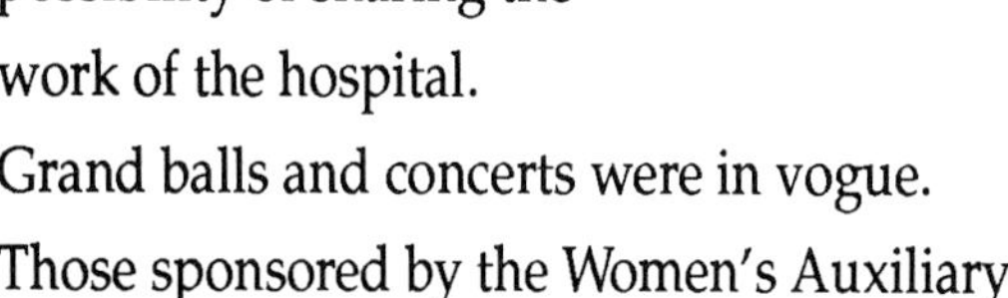

Grand balls and concerts were in vogue. Those sponsored by the Women's Auxiliary constituted some of the most stately and artistic attractions recorded in Chicago's social calendar. One of the more significant was the benefit concert of June 16, 1909 at the Auditorium Theatre. Chaired by Mrs. George R. Mueller, it included prominent Chicago vocalists Harriet M. Smulski, Rose K. Kwasigroch, Rose Olitzka, the Paulist Choir and the Philharmonic Orchestra.

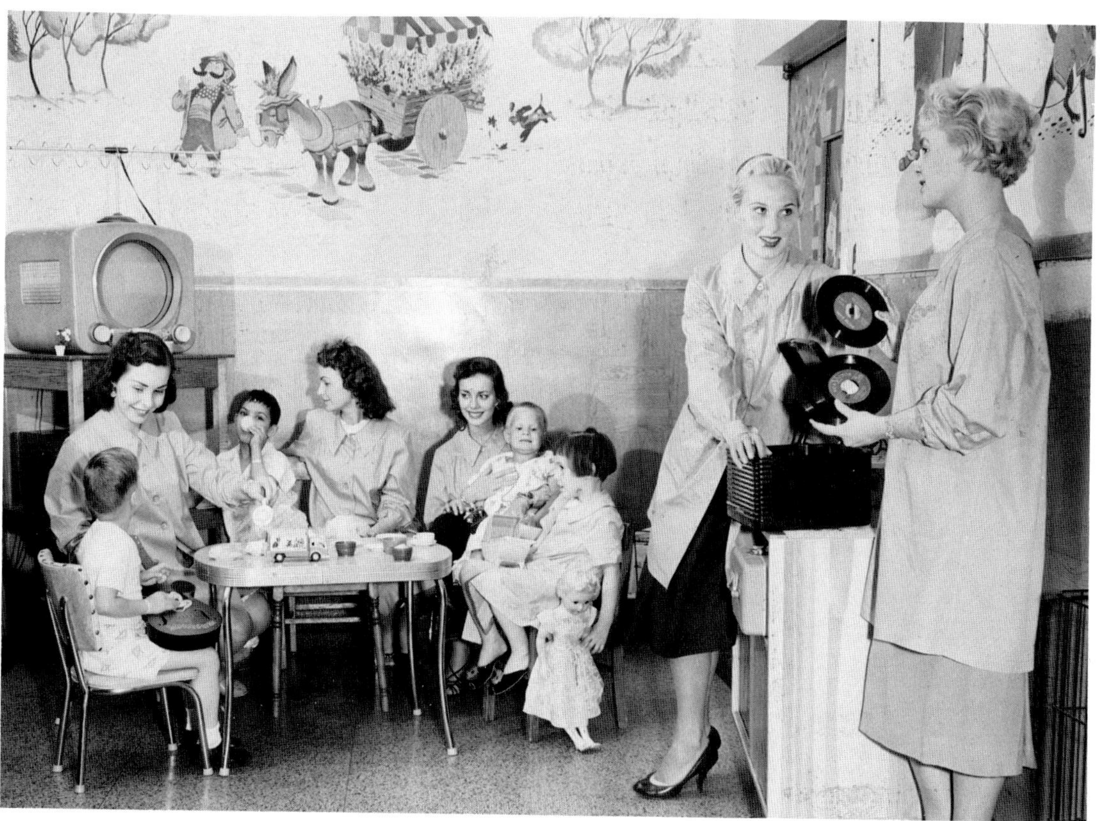

Members of the Women's Auxiliary with pediatric patients, 1950s

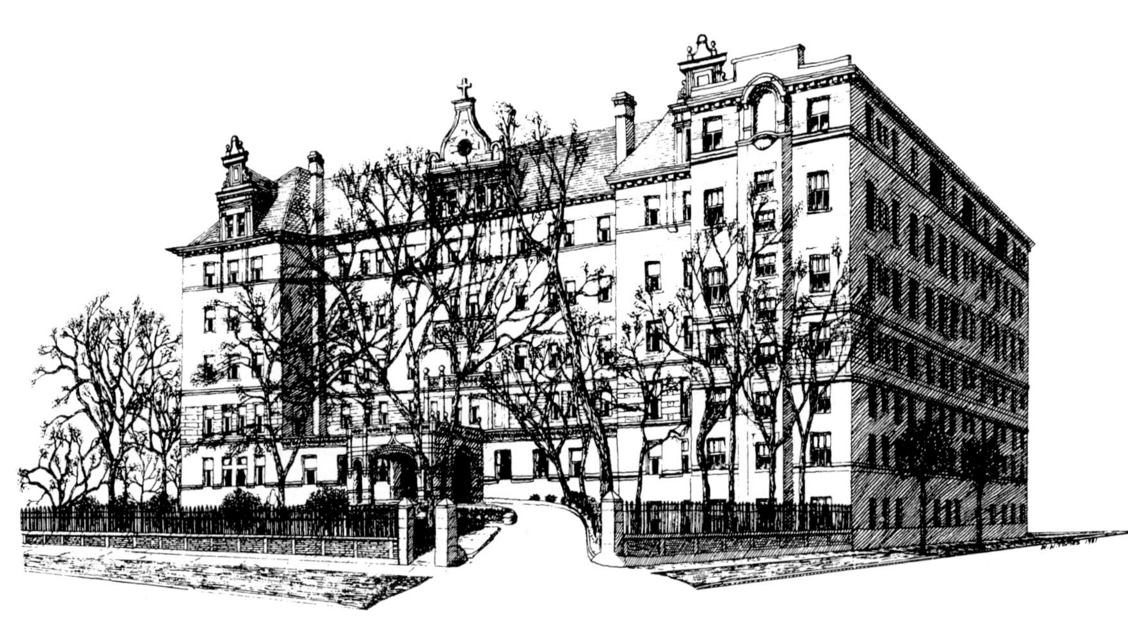

CHAPTER II

The Pride of Polonia Chicagoska

As the reputation of the hospital continued to spread, admissions kept growing. It became apparent that a new and much larger structure was needed. Mother Frances and the governing board approved a plan to build a $260,000 building on a square-block site bounded by Haddon Street and Oakley Boulevard, and Leavitt and Thomas Streets.

To gather ideas and opinions from experts on hospital design and construction, Dr. Ochsner, Mother Lauretta and architect Henry J. Schlack visited hospitals across the country. They had decided to incorporate the latest concepts into the new hospital before formal planning began. One feature on which they insisted was an absolutely fireproof building.

The plans were presented by the architect after he made independent visits to several of the best eastern hospitals. His investigations resulted in many modern improvements.

When the foundation was being laid, the October 27, 1900, edition of *Dzienik Chicagoska* described the new hospital in glowing detail: "The front of this beautiful edifice will be turned (east) towards Leavitt Street, separated from the street by 150 feet in order that the turmoil, noise, and dust will not enter it. The wards will be wide and light and will have six beds; the private rooms will be comfortably arranged. There will be operating rooms, baths, a physical therapy room and the reading room (library). On every floor there will be lovely verandas, as well as a large reception room for receiving people who would like advice or medical help from the doctors. In a word," the newspaper continued, "this hospital, as to its architectural design as well as its interior organization, will be a first-class hospital in the city and will become the pride of Polonia Chicagoska."

In one of her letters to Mother

Frances, Mother Lauretta expressed some doubts about the new institution. Knowing Mother Frances' love of poverty and simplicity, Mother Lauretta thought that the hospital was too large and too expensive. The loving and compassionate Foundress reassured her spiritual daughter in these comforting words: "Why do you fear that I should find the hospital too imposing, too large? I know well enough that it would have been impractical to construct a smaller building at this time. I trust you have a sufficient number of Sisters to staff it, and may their work in the spirit of sacrifice and dedication glorify God."

Greatly relieved with the understanding and consoling response, Mother Lauretta continued to supervise the work, seeing that the workers adhered conscientiously to the approved blueprints.

Cornerstone celebration

The ceremonial laying of the cornerstone was on June 16, 1901. What an event it must have been! At four o'clock in the afternoon, Building Commissioner Peter Kiolbassa, chief marshal of the day, led 4,000 men of the various Catholic societies, Polish predominating, to the hospital. In

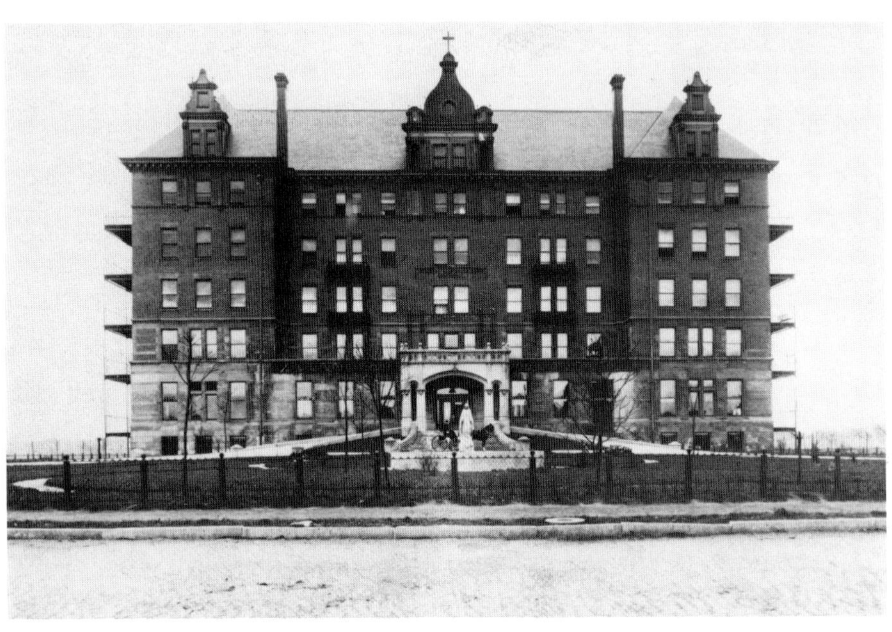

Saint Mary's, 1120 North Leavitt Street, soon after completion, 1903
(photo courtesy of the Chicago Historical Society)

this line were a troop of Polish cavalry, St. Stanislaus cadets, Polish Hussars of St. Adalbert's, St. Joseph Society, Holy Trinity Society, Polish Turners and Polish Foresters.

An article in *The Chicago Illinois News* for June 15, 1901, explained that Archbishop Feehan had a heavy schedule of pastoral duties for Sunday, June 16: three new Roman Catholic institutions, two churches and one new hospital to be blessed. Therefore, he appointed the Very Reverend Abbot N. Jaeger, OSB, abbot of the Benedictine monastery, to officiate at the 3:30 p.m. ceremony of laying the cornerstone at the new hospital. Pope Leo XIII dispatched a cablegram with his apostolic blessing.

Without fanfare, the name changed from Holy Family of Nazareth to Saint Mary of Nazareth Hospital.

The modern, professionally planned building was ready for occupancy, and the doors opened March 12, 1902. Dedicated by the Auxiliary Bishop of Chicago, Most Reverend Peter J. Muldoon, DD, High Mass was celebrated by Reverend Casimir Slominski, rector of St. Ann's Church. On March 18, under the

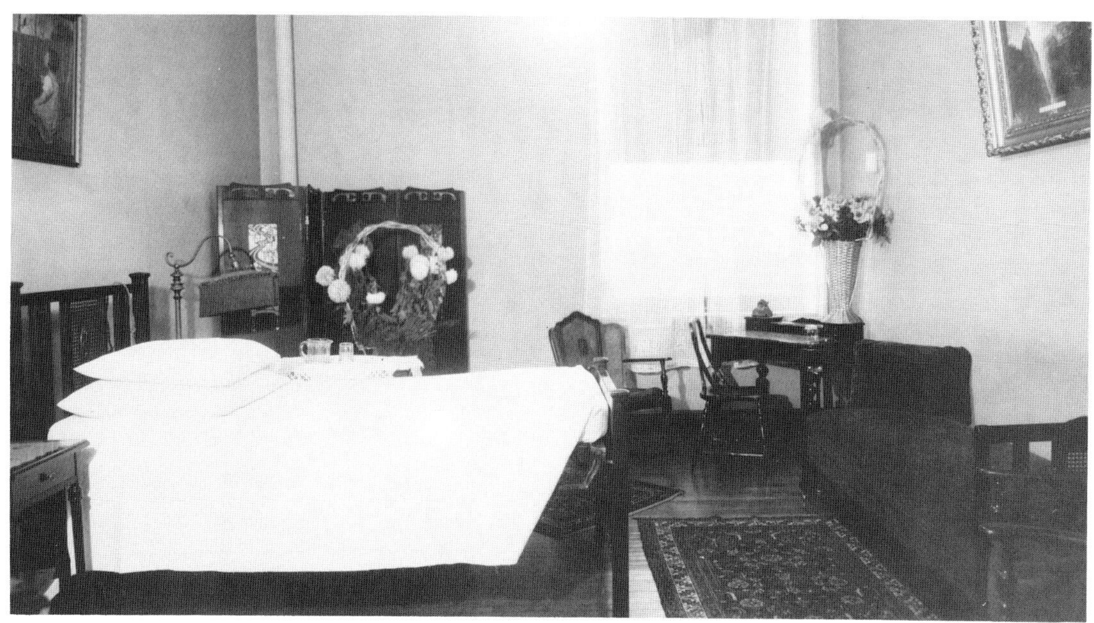

A private patient room, 1904

supervision of Hospital Director Sister Mary Donata Mindak and the physicians, patients were moved to the new hospital. The following day, fittingly on the feast of St. Joseph, Mass was celebrated for the first time in the beautiful Renaissance chapel.

The 25-year anniversary album informs the reader: "The location of the hospital is ideal in that it is located in a quiet residential neighborhood and removed from traffic and car lines. No high buildings or factories obstruct the view, and the patients daily enjoy the panorama of the northwest section of the city, which greets the eye from the upper verandas. These conveniences and delightful surroundings aid the patients materially in forgetting their helpless condition and seemingly endless hours of wearying idleness. The patients have the use of a garden in the rear of the hospital building containing approximately 42,000 square feet. For the special benefit of convalescent patients there are large porches on both north and south wings, where they may enjoy the fresh air." These large, enclosed porches off each floor on the north and south of the building were 12 feet by 55 feet and could be enclosed in winter.

Over the next 73 years, Saint Mary's would undergo 13 major renovations and additions,

Daytime surgery

The new Saint Mary's had other notable features. At the turn of the century, hospital floors were rarely stacked on top of one another. Buildings of one or two stories were the norm. This 297-bed hospital rose to five stories and included an outpatient emergency room and an X-ray room. It was a building "built to be a hospital." There was no modern air conditioning, so each story was about 17 feet high.

Dr. Albert Ochsner designed the operating rooms. On the top floor on the north, the principal surgery room measured over 24 feet square and was 18 feet high. It had one large window eight by 24 feet, and a skylight. Otherwise, the room was entirely bare, with white walls and ceiling, glazed tile and the floor in white

References to trees appear several times in chronicles, descriptions and activities of the hospital history. An example from the 1919 Silver Jubilee album: 'If 25 years ago our community of hospital workers was a weak twig transplanted to this country, and if today we see this twig grown to a strong tree, this has undoubtedly been accomplished only by the charitable cooperation of our friends and benefactors, and also by the indefatigable cooperation of the clergy, the respected doctors on our staff, and worthy members of the Women's Auxiliary. To each and every one we owe our most heartfelt thanks.'

— the Sisters of the Holy Family of Nazareth

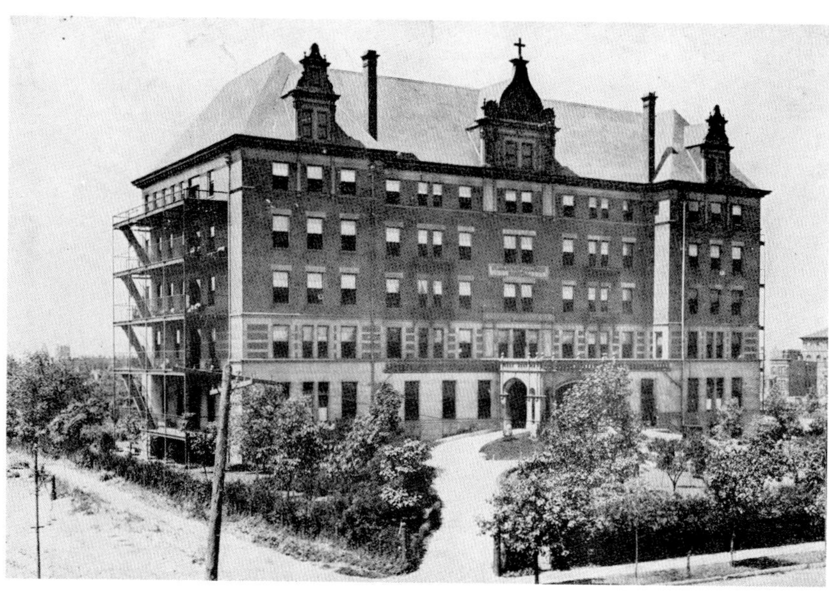

Early view of Saint Mary of Nazareth Hospital, showing porches

vitreous tile. Dr. Ochsner selected the top floor to take advantage of the skylights. When the hospital opened, there was some gaslight, but electricity would not be installed until 1914. There was truth to the admonition that if one needed surgery, they'd best need it during daylight hours. The surgeons rarely operated at night.

In her book *Out of Nazareth*, Sister Mary De Chantal, CSFN, reported that "the solemn public dedication was performed on May 25, 1902, with the participation of the clergy and the leading civic groups."

Immediately upon opening, there was an influx of patients; not only Polish immigrants but people of all religions and nationalities were admitted.

Her final reward

Her intense labors had gradually drained the strength of Mother Frances. She had scarcely recovered from a serious illness when she began to work again. Under the strain of her superhuman efforts, she finally succumbed—just eight months after the dedication of the new hospital.

Mother Cecilia attended to Mother Frances' needs in her final days. She bent over her and whispered that Mother Frances should take her to heaven along with her. The Foundress looked at her with a steadfast gaze, shook her head, and said in a thoughtful and solemn voice: "No. Lauretta. Lauretta . . . remain for her." Her last words, in a whisper, were "Jesus, Mary, Joseph." Mother Frances, known to her Sisters as Mother Mary of Jesus, the Good Shepherd, died in Rome on the feast of the Presentation of Mary, Friday, November 21, 1902.

"Our Mother Foundress is called the Saint of Division Street," Saint Mary's President Sister Stella Louise said recently, "because she walked through these streets. She founded this hospital. She spoke four or five languages, so she was able to relate to many groups of people. She was tireless. An example of her humanity: when she was on the ship going back to Rome, she took time to tutor a group of sailors. She was lamented not only by her 291 Sisters in 29 houses on both sides of the Atlantic, but also by all who knew her."

My mother began cleaning office buildings downtown, and continued in that work for many years. Life was physically difficult then, but we had good times, too. On Saturday afternoons, we scrubbed our white wooden floors, in our fourth floor walkup, and spread newspapers over them so they'd be clean for Sunday. On Sunday, we did as little work as possible: we dressed up to go to church, and we stayed dressed up all day. Sometimes we went to Lincoln Park or to social club dances in the evening. Most of the married women worked outside their homes. It wasn't considered unusual, and certainly no one thought that the children were being neglected. The Poles in my neighborhood didn't have much to do with people of other nationalities. They believed in staying within one's own group, and especially, marrying within that group. Once an Italian boy came to pick me up at my home; my parents were deeply shocked that I could even consider him as a date. All our neighbors were Polish, and most were immigrants. Almost everyone was happy to be here.

We were a lot happier with less then than we are with more now.'

The Great Depression

When the economic crisis of the 1930s swept the nation, it defeated the charitable nature of many hospitals. Sustaining funds were lacking when they were in greatest demand. Charity services were curtailed. It required deep sympathy to forget one's own difficulties and show hospitality to numerous indigent patients. While Saint Mary's finances were so strained, it required shrewd business tactics to retain the creditors' goodwill—and strong faith to carry on. The optimism of Superintendent Sister Mary Basilla Frelich was equal to the task.

In an interview with Sacred Heart Province historian Sister Mary Edith Willow, CSFN, PhD, Sister Virtunia Chmura said: "I came to Saint Mary's Hospital on August 28, 1930, after pronouncing my perpetual vows. ... We worked 12 to 14 hours in the hospital, and then did our housework and cooking in the convent, too. Those were hard years, but most of us enjoyed the work and have no regrets. In 1930, we had 114 Sisters here to share the work and the good times, too."

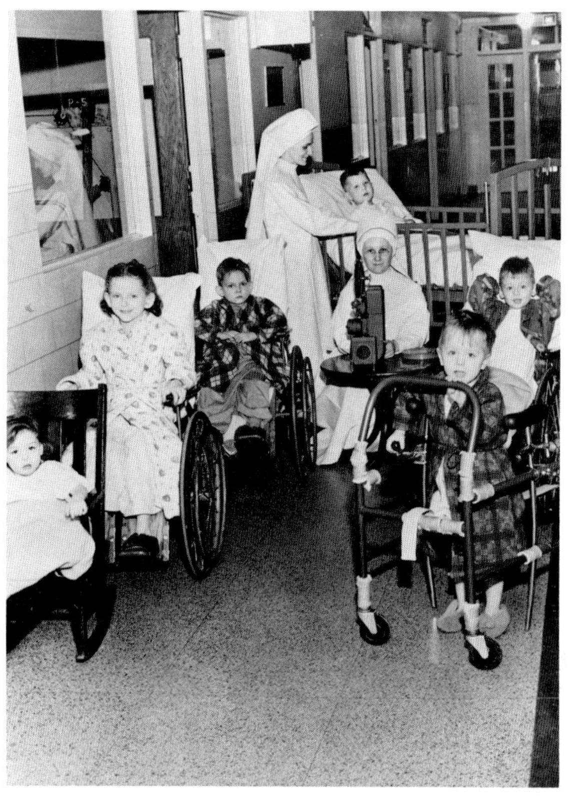

Sister Virgil at projector, and Sister Alphonsa, standing, with pediatric patients

The Depression and recovery years, although severe and debilitating, had a salutary effect on Saint Mary's. Blue Cross and pre-payment health plans that were inaugurated during the Depression stabilized hospital income to some degree and, as Sister Virtunia said, "made it possible to think of budgets with greater confidence."

The Junior Auxiliary

The 1944, 50th anniversary book describes the energetic Junior Auxiliary: 'By the time the administration of the hospital reached the decision, in 1930, to extend the facilities by a north wing, a new ally had been acquired—the Junior Auxiliary, organized by Mrs. L. Dyniewicz, a prominent member of the senior association.'

'Armed,' as the album states, 'with zestful initiative and imagination, their sympathy for the hospital's aims proved richly productive from the very outset.' Their fundraising efforts, at least in the beginning, centered on maintenance and modernization of the X-ray equipment. 'Their monthly meetings are powerfully charged with vitality and appreciation of timely issues,' the book continues. 'Their annual charity affair is always a fitting tribute to the motives which gave rise to the organization.'

Hospital admissions fell in the early 1930s, but in 1934 they started to rise again.

Monsignor John Mecikowski, Saint Mary's chaplain for 32 years, shared some of his reminiscences in 1960. When he arrived in 1932, he found 152 Sisters working as elevator operators, telephone operators, and in various departments of the hospital, as well as at the bedsides of patients. They did all of the manual work done by the lay personnel today. He reported that "the doctors never—or very seldom—operated on any person who was past 60 years of age. Patients stayed several weeks in the hospital, and today they usually go home after one week."

During the years 1937-44, the medical staff made a concerted effort to improve the quality of education it provided to its interns. Saint Mary's joined other Chicago hospitals in offering each intern additional course work and lectures by various staff doctors in their areas of specialty. Doctors Larkowski, Steinert and Warszewski, surgeons and instructors,

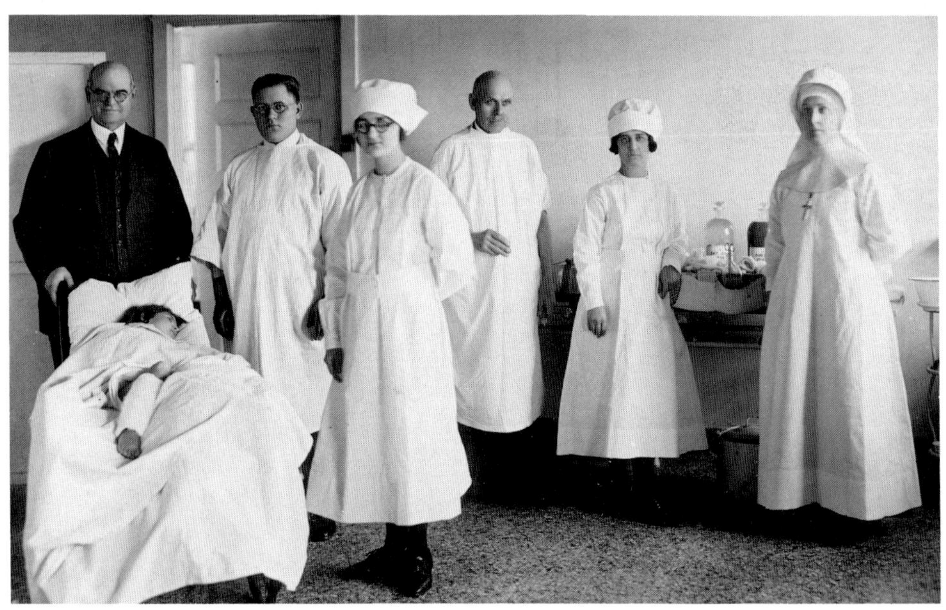

On the left, Dr. George Mueller, Chief of the Medical Staff from 1937-43, and Dr. Thaddeus Larkowski, Chief of Staff from 1943-50

worked especially hard to improve the interns' education program by providing more intensive instruction. They established rotations to assure that each intern gained experience in the major clinical services.

The Global War

When America went to war again in 1941, the hospital staff had to relearn how to provide uninterrupted healthcare to the community with fewer supplies and qualified personnel. In whatever way they could, those who remained did their best to contribute to the war effort.

In the early years of the war, the possibility of enemy air attack was very real. All hospitals were asked to be prepared to give aid in the event of attack. The Sisters equipped the operating rooms to handle three major operations under total blackout conditions. Saint Mary's became so proficient in blacking itself out

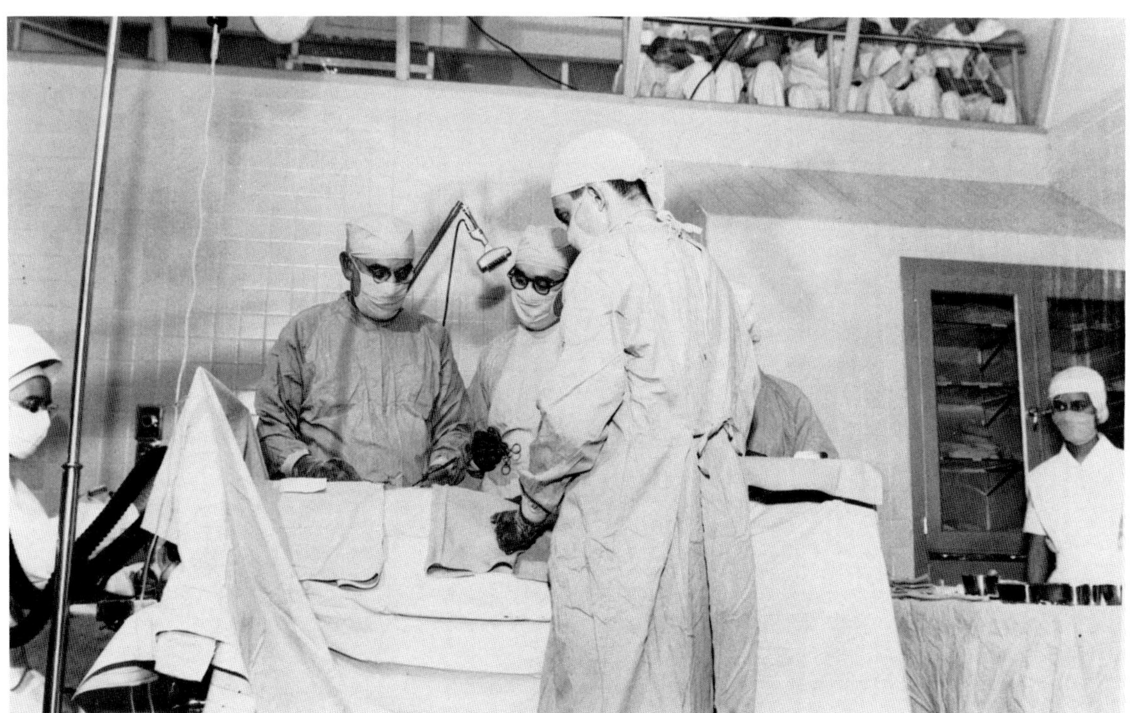

Operating room with observation balcony, Leavitt Street hospital, circa 1945

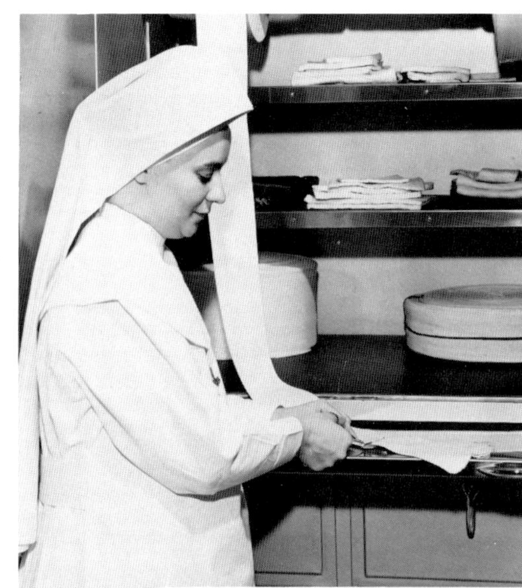

Sister Honesta,
orthopedics room,
circa 1945

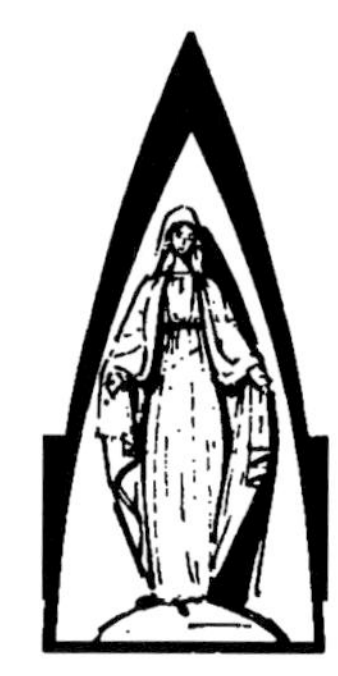

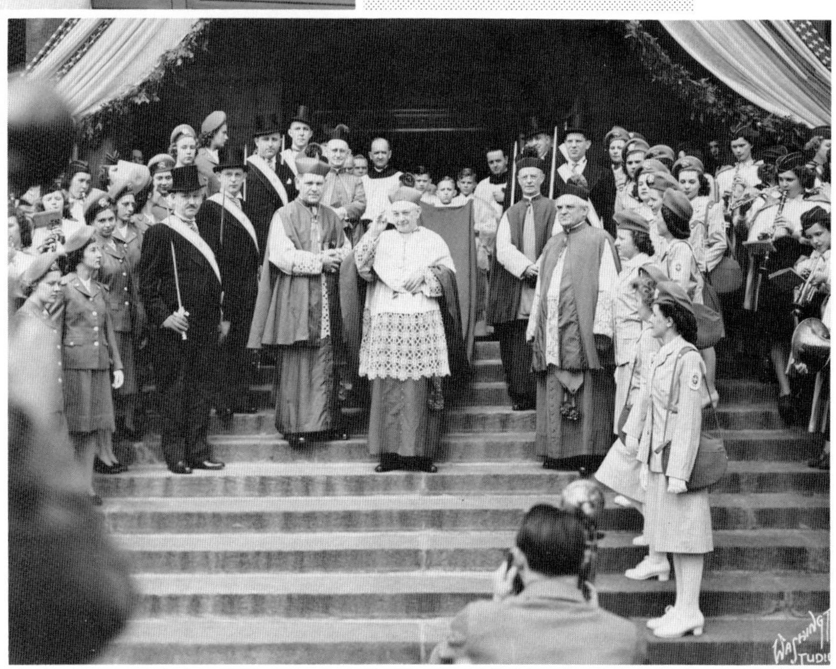

The Golden Jubilee of Saint Mary's was celebrated with members of the U.S. Nurse Cadet Corps and the Holy Family Academy Band. Church officials in attendance included, from left, Monsignor Strzycki, Bishop Bona, Cardinal Stritch, Monsignor Rusch and Monsignor Ostrowski.

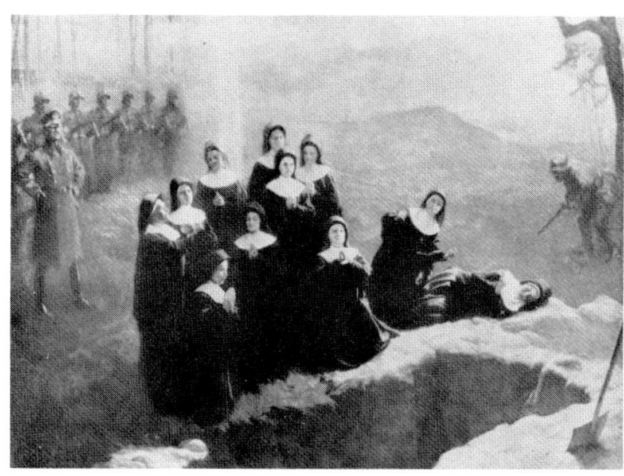

The Martyred Sisters of the Holy Family of Nazareth, 1943

In 1943 Poland was in the darkest period of Nazi occupation. In Nowogrodek, 12 Sisters of the Holy Family of Nazareth shared the fear of their neighbors. They sympathized with those who were under arrest, detained in concentration camps, or doomed to execution. The Sisters, although restricted in their apostolic endeavors, continued serving the people of God as they could.

After witnessing the arrest of men in their neighborhood, Sister Stella Mardosewicz, the Superior, expressed to Father Aleksander Zienkiewicz the Sisters' wish in this prayer: "O God, if sacrifice of life is needed, accept it from us who are free from family obligations. Spare those who have wives and children."

On July 31, 1943, 11 Sisters were arrested. The other Sister was elsewhere doing hospital work. In the early hours of August 1, after a night of imprisonment that is still shrouded in mystery, the Sisters were packed into a van and driven beyond the town's limits. They were shot and placed in a common grave in a wooded area. Subsequently, the death sentences of the most recently arrested men in Nowogrodek were commuted; some were released and permitted to return home, while others were sent off to perform hard labor.

After the Nazis left, the bodies of the Sisters were exhumed. The grateful people of Nowogrodek honored the Sisters in a solemn funeral service. They were given proper burial in a cemetery adjoining the local church.

Perhaps the motto of the Sisters of the Holy Family offers some insight:
"Behold, the Kingdom of
God is within you."

that it offered detailed instructions to other hospitals so that they, too, would be better prepared to avert any possible attack.

Supplies and staff became scarcer as the war continued. Out of necessity, doctors volunteered to teach the Sister supervisors and nurses how to administer intravenous fluids and give blood transfusions. That was considered so radical then that the doctors had to assume supervisory responsibility, in the event of any legal action taken against them.

Fifty-five physicians and 49 nurses left the hospital for the armed forces. Even with so many people on active duty here and abroad, patient admissions continued to climb. Critically short of nurses, workloads for remaining nurses nearly doubled. The number of student nurses and interns declined, and in 1942 there were no interns at all. Sisters and nurses assumed new tasks previously performed

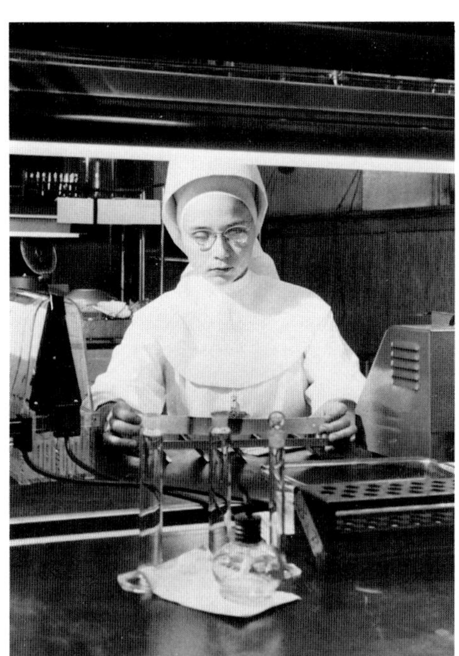

Laboratory, 1940s

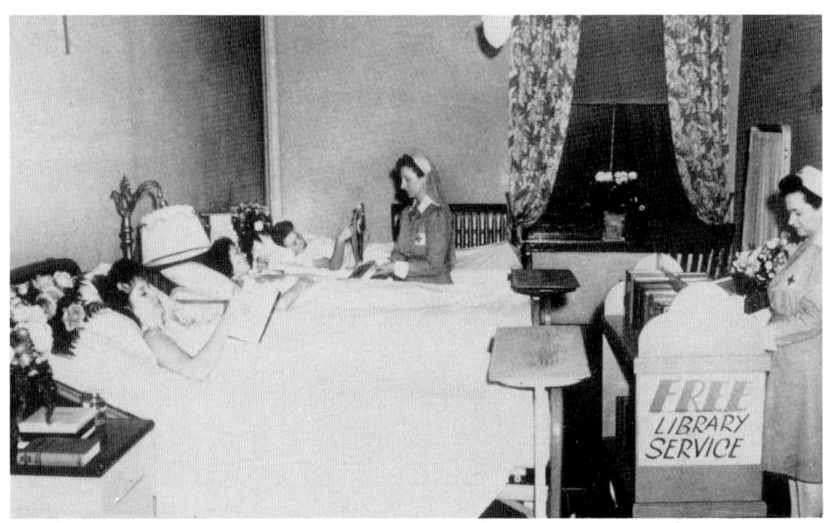

Red Cross Volunteers

Nursery, 1940s

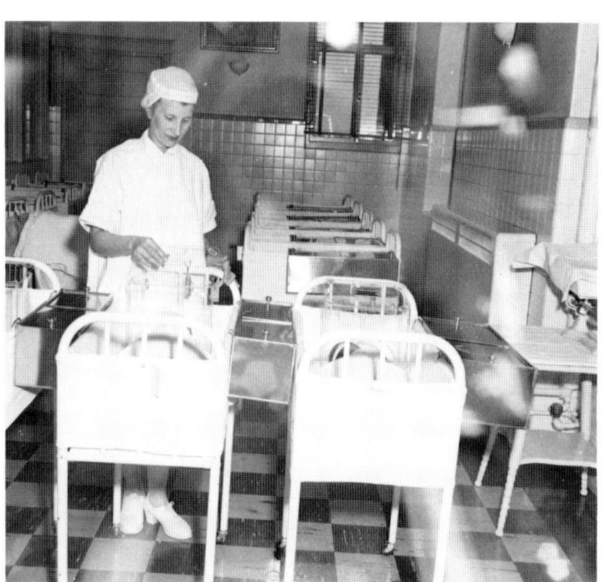

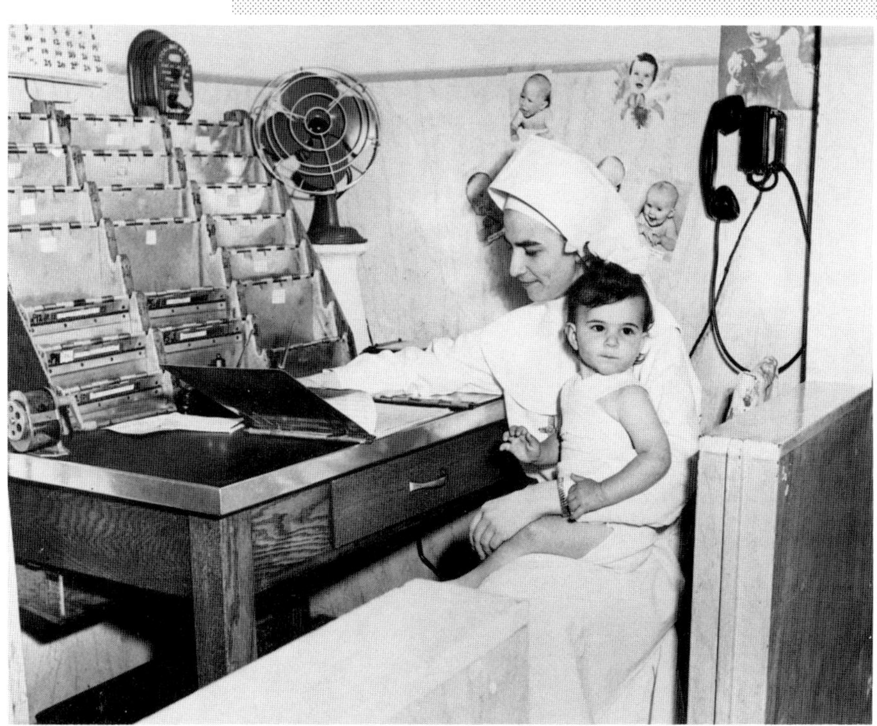

Sister Bernadette in pediatrics chart room, circa 1945

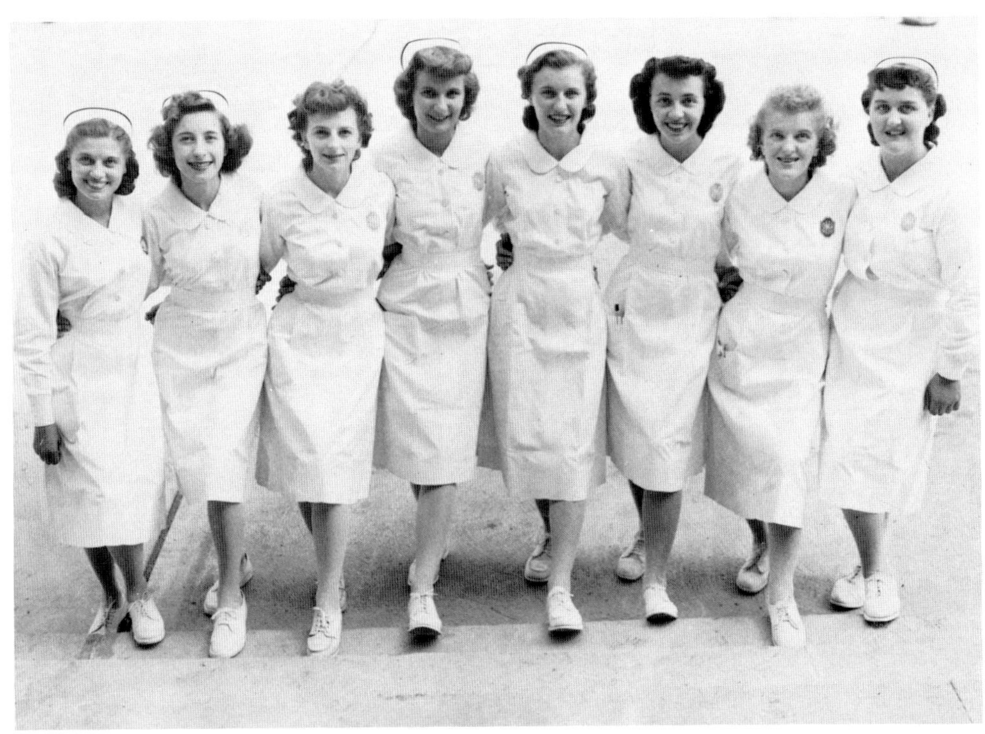

Two of these eight student nurses would represent Weber and Holy Trinity High Schools when the two football teams met at Soldier Field on Sunday, September 19, 1948, in the second annual charity game for the benefit of the nurses building fund. From left to right are: Theresa Grembla, Vivian Florio, Adeline Stefanowski, Dorothy Rzasa, Teresa Koziol, Mayme Ferratto, Genevieve Gall and Helen Koch.

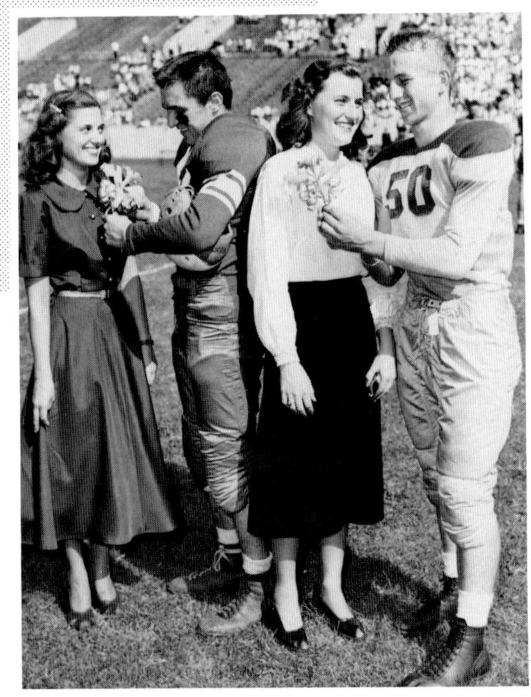

The winning nurses, Theresa Grembla and Teresa Koziol

exclusively by doctors.

The Women's Auxiliary met regularly at the hospital to knit and sew bandages and clothing. To offset the loss of medical personnel called into service, the hospital opened American Red Cross classes in first aid and home nursing. The Sisters not only enrolled in the first class but also let the Red Cross use their hospital to conduct classes. (The affiliation continues to this day: the Red Cross conducts CPR classes at the hospital.)

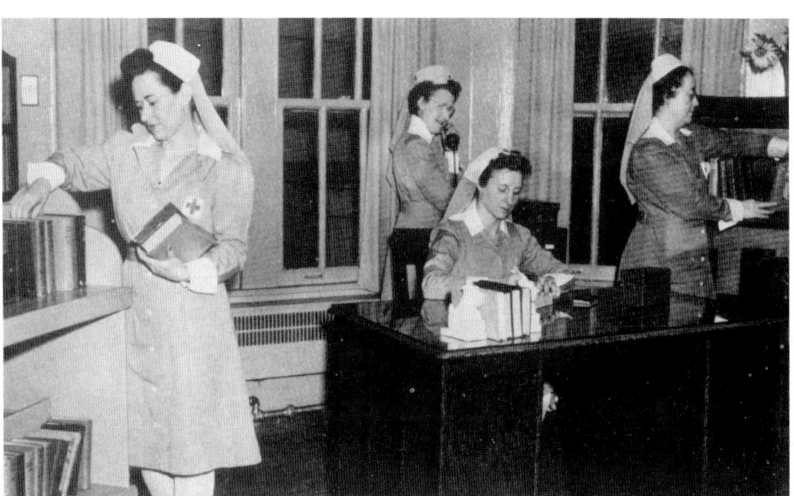
Gray Ladies created the patient library.

Almost immediately after the outbreak of war, friends of the hospital appeared, offering to help and devoting many hours to a variety of tasks. Homemakers and business and professional women volunteered. Nurses' aides who had completed Red Cross courses helped relieve the overworked staff. A corps of Gray Ladies, wearing distinctive gray uniforms with a red cross emblem and a small white headdress, rendered invaluable assistance in the admitting and Nursing School offices.

By changing some services that nurses traditionally performed to meet wartime realities, the hospital managed to carry on during the conflict.

A cablegram arrived during Saint Mary's Golden Jubilee in 1944: "With deep joy we give recognition to the praiseworthy record which the Sisters of the Holy Family of Nazareth have established in their sublime mission, for we are not unaware of the devoted, self-sacrificing, humanitarian labors emanating from that indefatigable Christian charity which constantly urges them on. ..."—Pope Pius XII

In the wake of war

At the end of 1944, the medical staff had 126 members; 41 Sisters were registered nurses. Patient admissions rose to 10,500; of these, 1,816 were newborn infants.

The war years brought economic and social changes to the neighborhood and to Saint Mary's. The predominance of Polish patients was giving way to many nationalities, just as

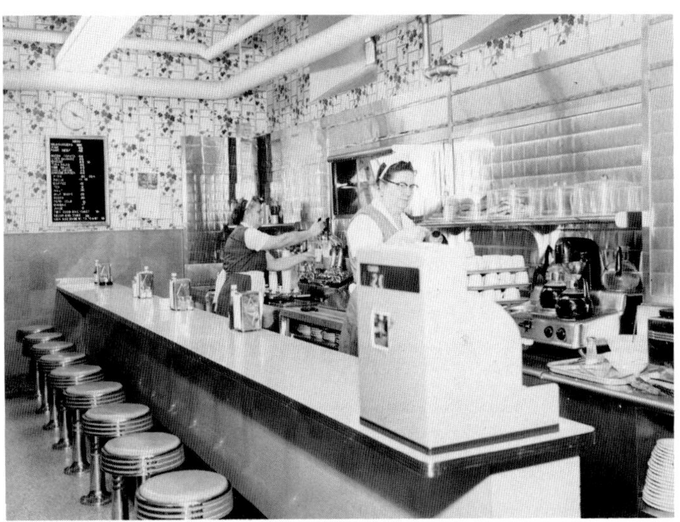

At the hospital snack shop in the 1950s, a cheeseburger was 30 cents, a sundae 17 cents and a Pepsi Cola ten cents.

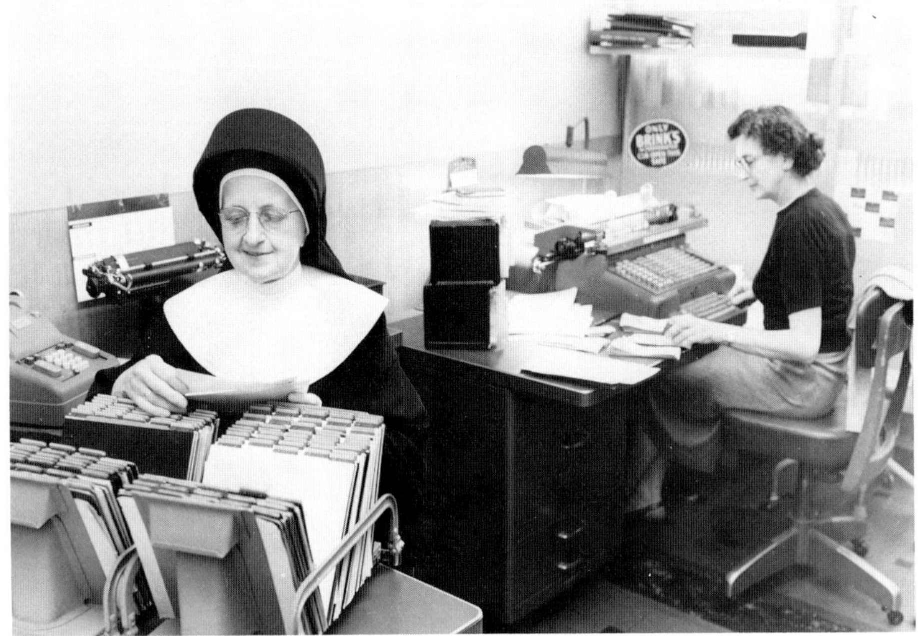

Sister M. Virtunia in the business office, 1950s

Unfortunately, the astronaunts' schedule could not accommodate the visit. So, according to C. Wayne Hamilton, currently vice president, corporate development and marketing, "We crashed the party at McCormick Place! We commandeered the Superior Coffee truck, emptied all the coffee out, and put this huge astro-birthday cake in the back of the truck. Sister Stella Louise and Sister Clemens got in and we went to McCormick Place. Because we were a delivery truck we got right through the Secret Service into the delivery docks, unloaded the cake, and wheeled it out onto the stage of the theater in front of 6,000 children from all over the city. Mayor Daley was there, and Vice President Humphrey. They looked around and here were two nuns coming out with this huge birthday cake in the shape of a

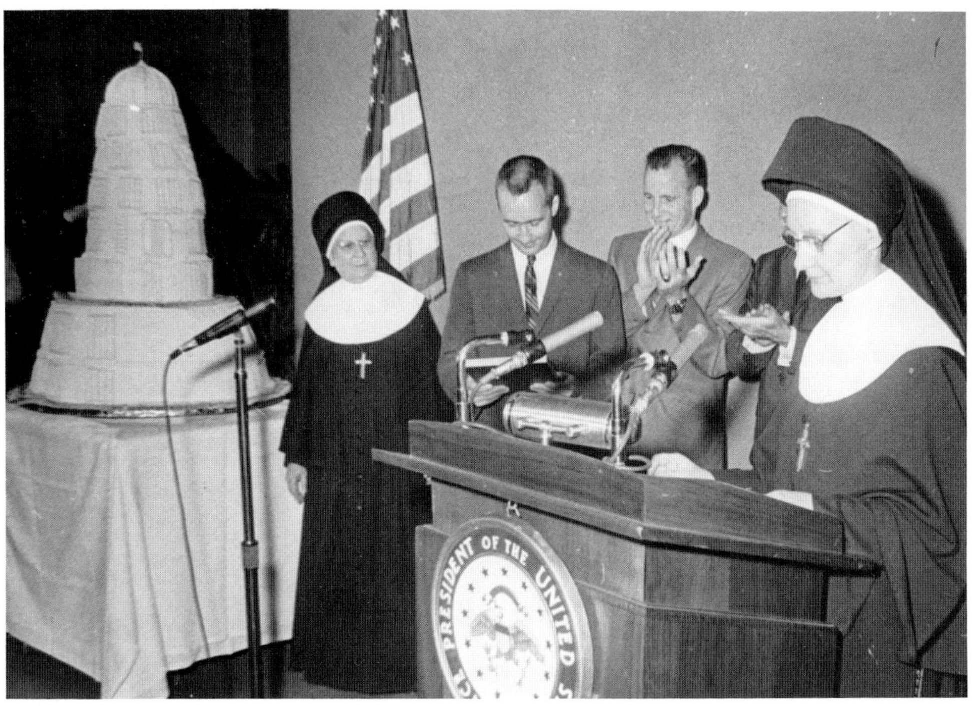

The finale of Astro-days at Saint Mary's, June 14, 1965. Sister Stella Louise has just presented plaques to astronauts McDivitt and White at McCormick Place. From left to right are: Sister Mary Clemens, Director of Social Service, astronaut James McDivitt, astronaut Edward White, and Sister Stella Louise. Vice President Hubert Humphrey and Chicago Mayor Richard J. Daley are behind Sister Stella Louise.

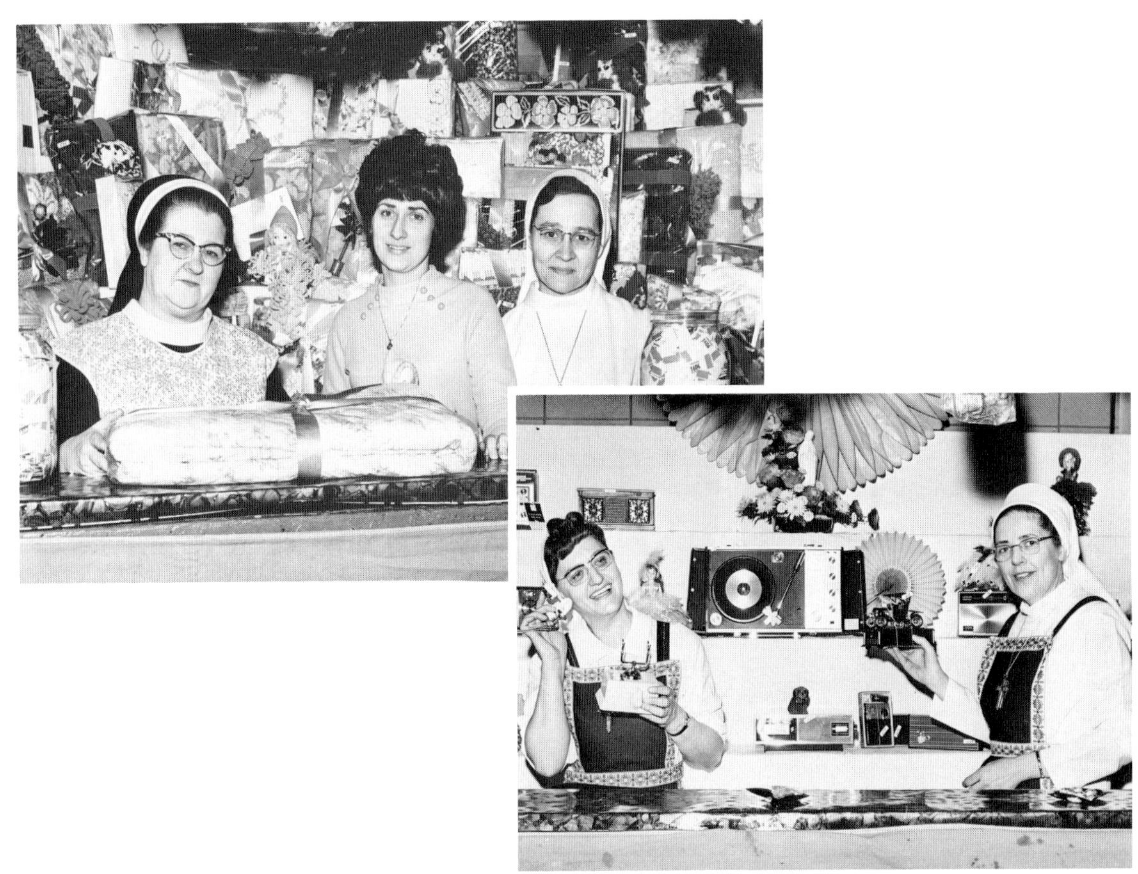

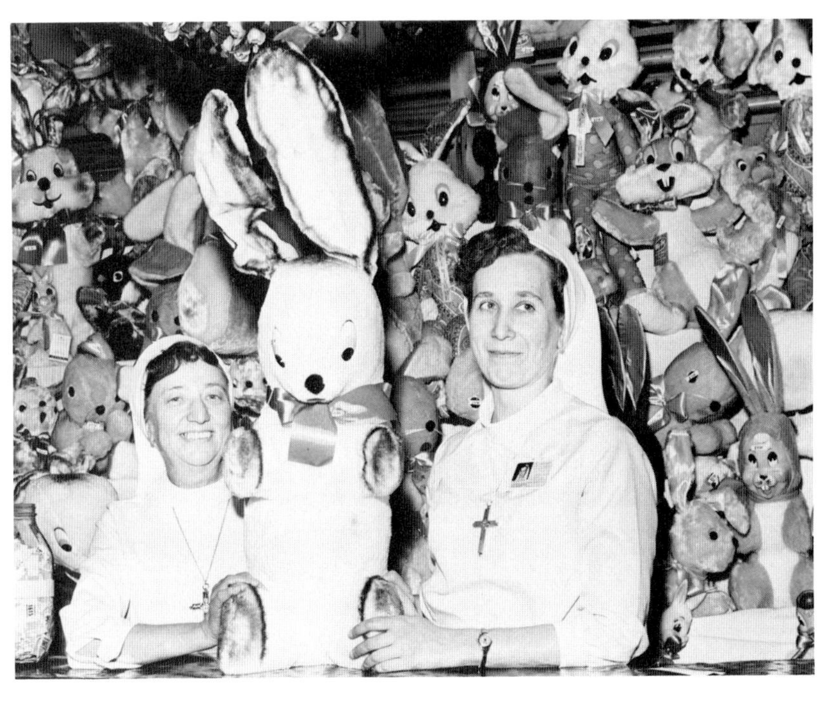

Hospital Bazaar,
March, 1970

ST. MARY OF NAZARETH HOSPITAL
PLANT YOUR MONEY
FREE ADMISSION
FESTIVAL
FRIDAY - MARCH 26 Noon - 11:00
SATURDAY - 27 3:00 - 11:00
SUNDAY - 28 Noon - 11:00
GYMNASIUM - 2255 West HADDON at OAKLEY
21" MAGNAVOX" COLOR T.V. RAFFLE PRIZES
Variety Booth
Radios - Recordings
Wallet - Purses

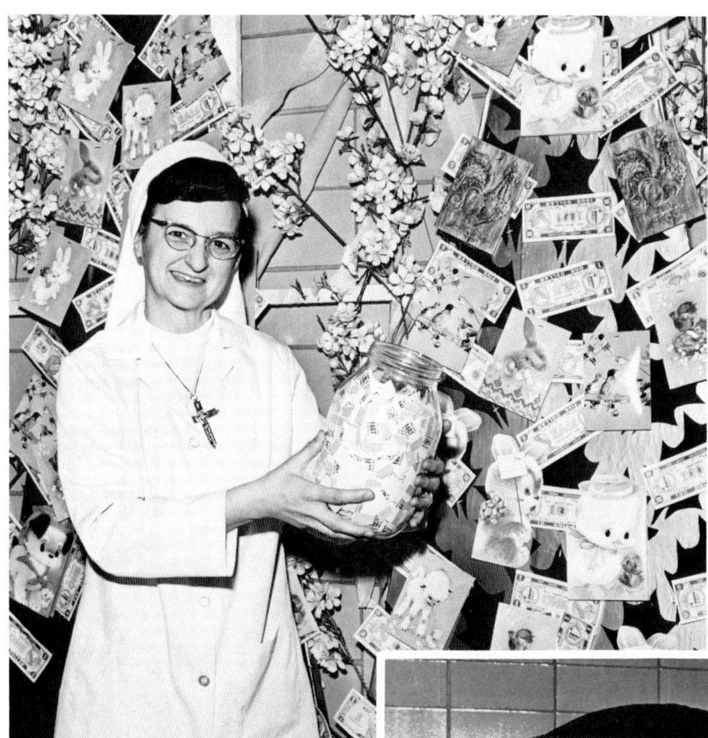

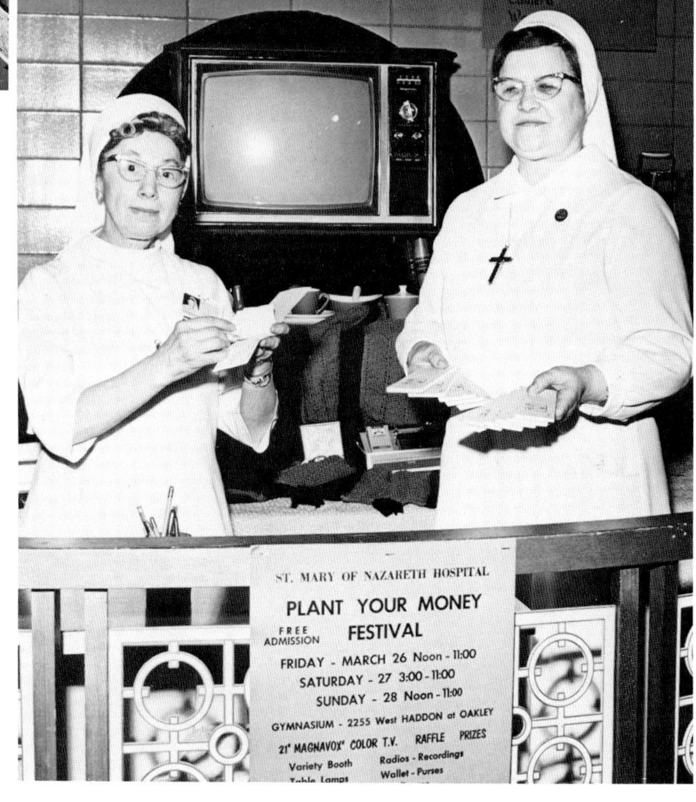

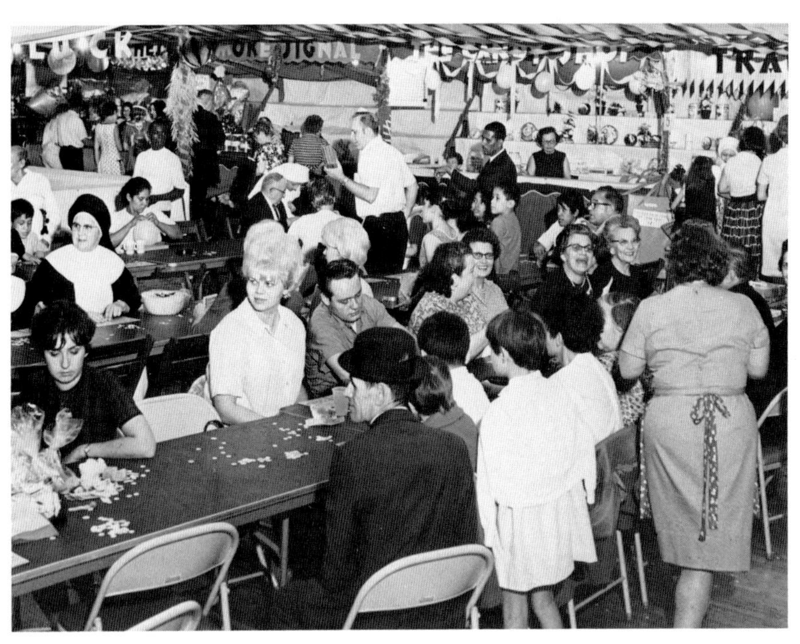

Hospital Bazaar, March, 1970

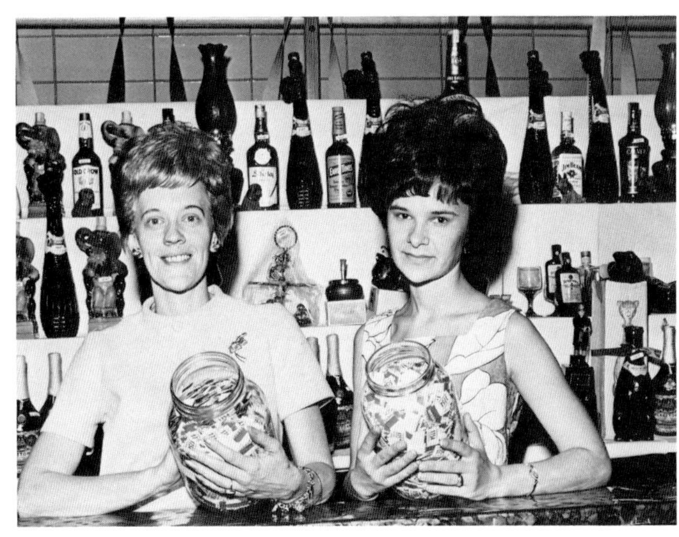

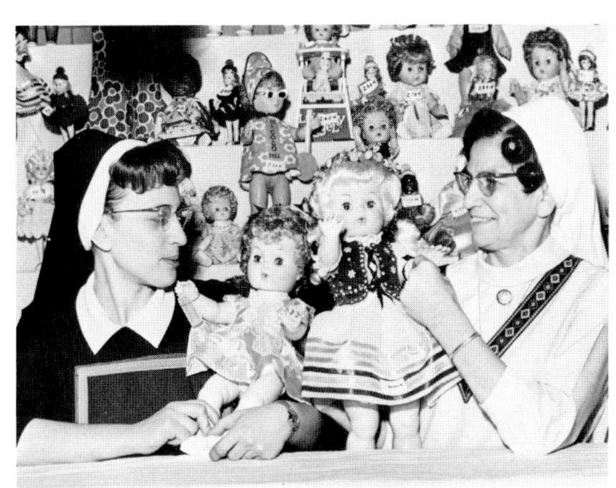

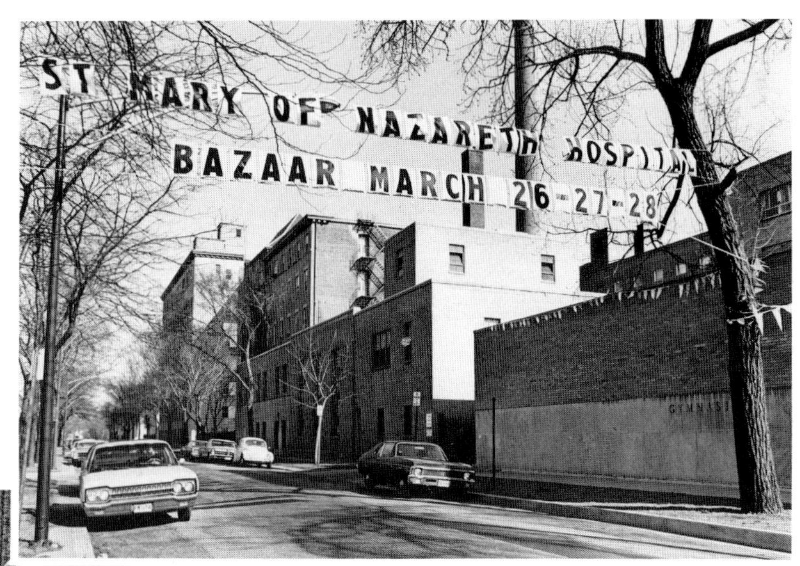
BAZAAR MARCH 26-27-28

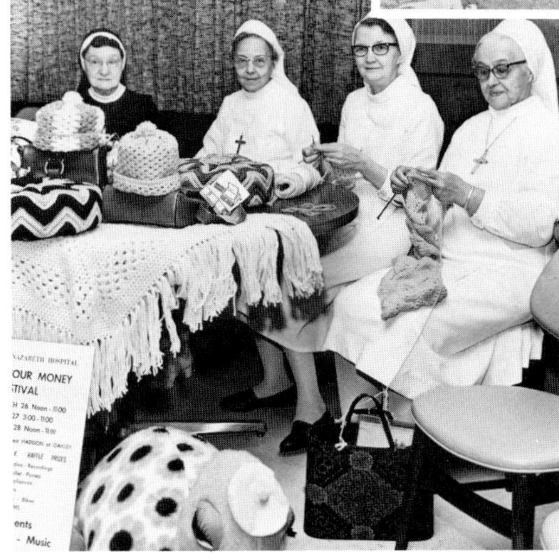
Music

space capsule. It tore up the house. At least we got his cake delivered."

Fifteen years later, McDivitt finally made it to the hospital. As Grand Marshall of the 1980 St. Patrick's Day Parade, he christened Saint Mary's float entry. Unfortunately, McDivitt cut his hand on the champagne bottle and needed a few stitches from the emergency department! The float won the first place award for community participation.

Convenience food

The first total "convenience food" dietary service in a Chicago hospital was started at Saint Mary's in 1967. It was born of necessity, and lasted over 20 years! When the hospital developed its structural split, the first thing that went was the kitchen. Wayne Hamilton, displaying his perpetual good humor, tells the story: "In the early 1960s we wondered—how were we going to do 2,000 meals a day with no kitchen? We went to a local delicatessen in the A&P supermarket on Chicago Avenue and asked them, Can you cut and wash lettuce, and make salads? Put them in plastic bags and potato chip tins?' We went to Armour and Swift. `Can you slice beef, cook it, cut it, roll it, freeze it with nitrogen gas, pre-portion it and sell it to us?' That was the beginning, at least in this area, of prepared convenience food. We sold all of our kitchen equipment. Our ovens went to a man who baked our potatoes for us. At first they tasted like cardboard. We discovered you have to extract a portion of the moisture before you bake a potato, or it gets dry and tastes like cardboard."

The completely pre-packaged, heat-and-serve food service operation drew considerable attention. Many manufacturers of electronic, mechanical and sophisticated engineering systems came to see the service in operation and offered research and development products and various other resources. A feature article in a 1967 issue of *Institutions Magazine* detailed Saint Mary's shift to "pre-prepared" patient foods, reheated for serving in microwave, infrared, steamer and convenience units, for both general and special diets. The cost savings and results: 75 percent reduction in production-labor outlays; 90 percent reduction in kitchen equipment expenses; 30 percent savings in space; instant upgrading of quality; dramatic reduction in overproduction; reduced shrinkage; and greater variety. Hamilton's research findings were published in various food trade journals, and *The Journal of the American Hospital Association* ran a feature article on this unique service.

1968 was the year Saint Mary's purchased neighboring Lutheran Deaconess Hospital (which moved to suburban Park Ridge as Lutheran General Hospital), and razed it to prepare a site for a new health center. It was also the year an Outpatient Mental Health Center was launched. One of the first such facilities, its emphasis was on the team approach, with a psychiatrist, psychologist and psychiatric social worker coordinating treatment.

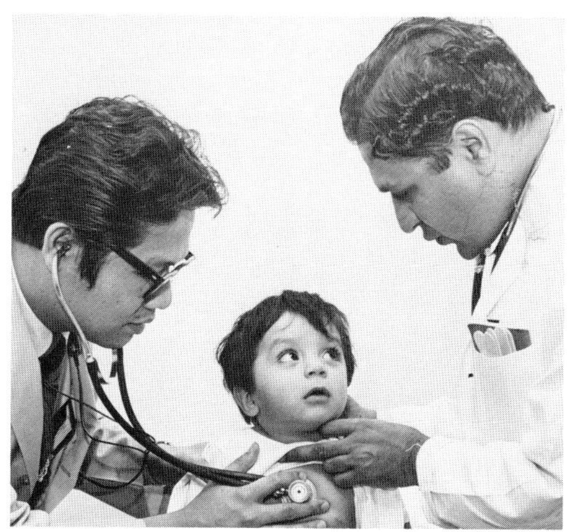

At left, Dr. Procopio Yanong examines a child during National Hospital Week, May 9-15, 1971.

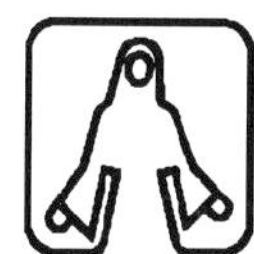

A new logo was adopted in 1970, which remains in use today. It portrays Mary of Nazareth with her hands outstretched—a graphic representation of how the hospital provides the greatest service possible to human beings through its concern and involvement in life. Sister Stella Louise said, "Its openness represents so beautifully and simply the completeness of dedication that is typical of Saint Mary's past, present, and the years to come."

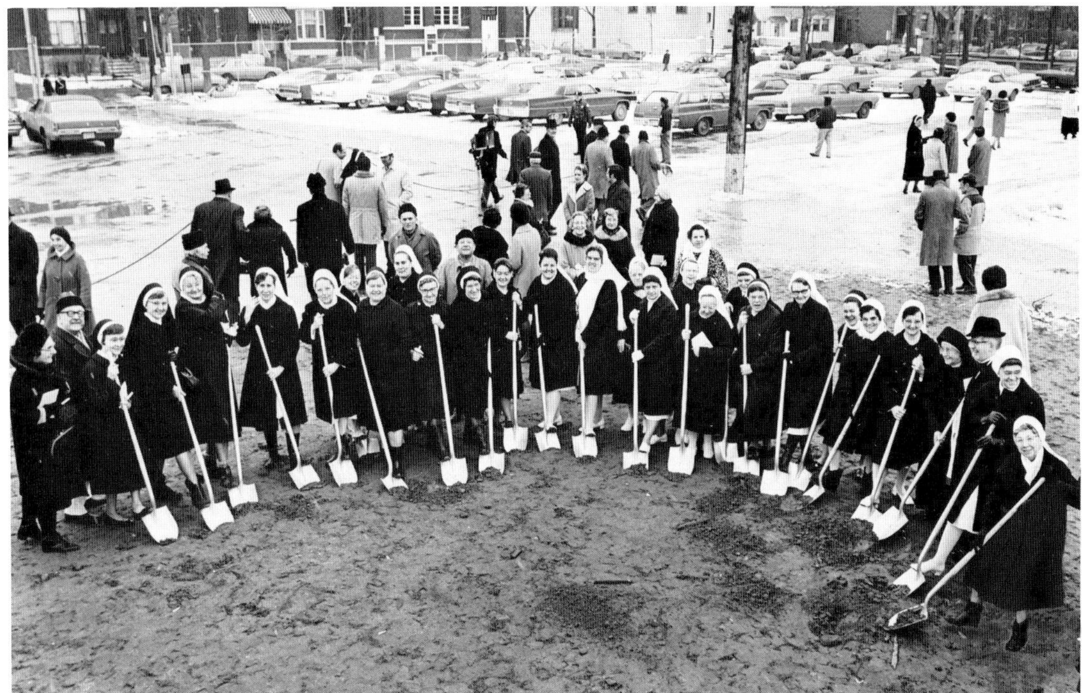

The Sisters gathered at the groundbreaking for the new hospital center.

Groundbreaking signals changes

When the groundbreaking ceremony took place on February 2, 1972, it was proclaimed that the new Hospital Center on Division and Leavitt Streets would be the first hospital in Illinois and one of the few in the world to have all single-bed patient rooms.

The Family Care Clinic opened in 1972 and became the setting for a new medical residency at Saint Mary's—the family practice residency. Located at 2238 West Thomas Street, the Family Care Clinic was designed to meet the healthcare needs of families without a regular physician.

Breaking up our house

Sophie Kass, RN, women's service coordinator, says, "I remember standing on the landing of the 5th floor fire escape of the old Saint Mary's, looking at this awesome gray structure growing out of the ground and thinking, `Oh great, now we will have the space we so desperately need. But how are we ever going to fill this huge complex?' I knew there would be new faces, new friendships, new challenges. But the old building had a sense of warmth, family and a sense of belonging, much like your own home does." Department of Nursing Staffing Coordinator Bernice Madaj, RN, agrees. She worked in the critical care area during the transition. "It was very exciting for us," she recalls. "There was a lot of new technology and we had more space. But there was also an element of isolation. For example, Central Supply used to be on the second floor nursing unit, and is now located on the lower level. And, we used to constantly see other employees as we ran up and down the open staircase. So people we used to see every day at least in passing we might not see for weeks at a time."

"You should have seen our chapel," says Sister Mary Bernadette, child life specialist. "It was like a cathedral! We had choir recitals and opera singers who said the acoustics were great. The hospital was like my own home, because I'd been in that home for 40 years ... I was nowhere else. It seemed like a part of me was taken away ... and when we saw it going down ... I was just crushed! I still yearn for the old building and for the people that were there and the things we used to do. The family atmosphere. We knew every doctor, every wife, every kid in their house. The kids used to come on Sundays and make rounds with their daddies to the patients. Very often we talk about it now. Something comes up and someone says, `Do you

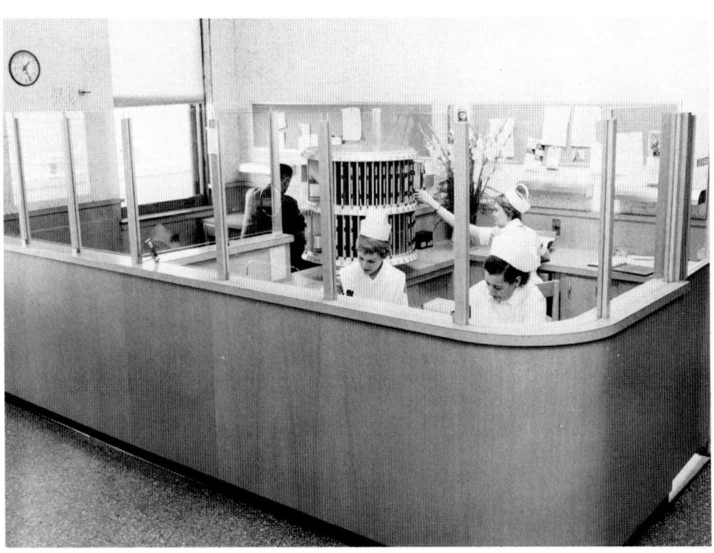

Nurses station, 1970

remember? ...' And then you go back, and you have such a soft spot. Oh, why did we ever knock it down? However, don't get me wrong. I love this place. I'd never want to change it. I'm all for change. But there was something ..."

George Mizia, director of security, was born at Saint Mary's. He married a graduate of the School of Nursing in 1977. Christine Mizia currently works at the hospital as well. George has some fond memories from his 24 years as an employee. "Sister Stella Louise wanted to learn to drive a car," he recalls. "This was in the old building. At that time the hospital had a '58 or '59 black Buick and she asked me to teach her how to drive. I would come in at seven o'clock and Sister and I would go to Humboldt Park and she would drive the car around. I don't know how many stop signs she drove through. She had a tendency of steering to the left. I kept saying to her, `To the right, to the right, to the right. ...' When she was doing better I

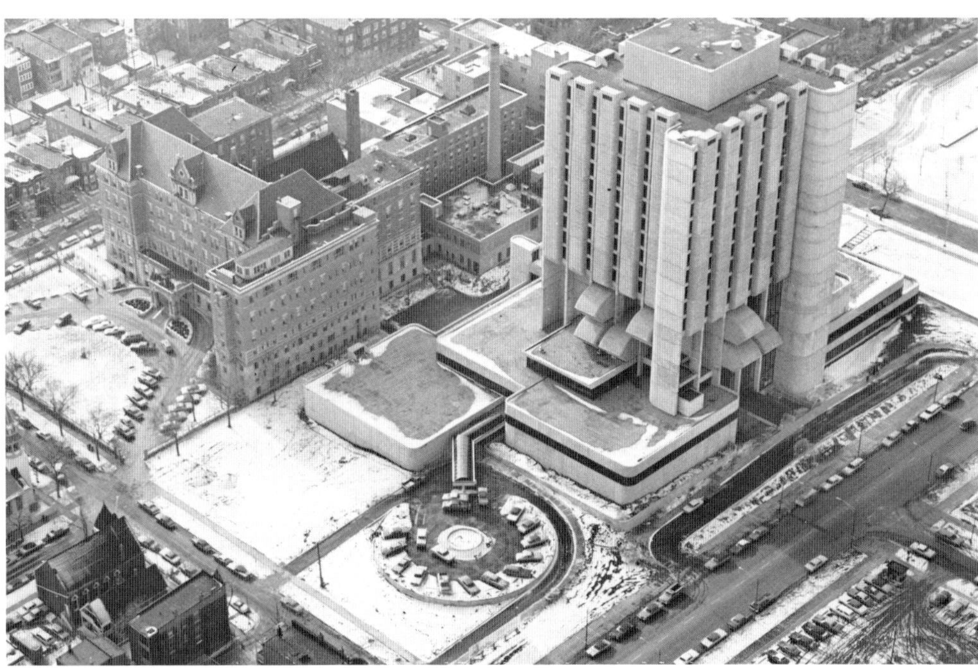

For a moment, both hospitals stood.

suggested that she go to a driving school. She did and subsequently got her license and now she's a real good driver. When she first asked me to take her out it was me making the sign of the cross before each excursion.

"One time—when patients could still smoke in their rooms—we got a fire alarm. The smell of smoke was traced to a patient room where oxygen had just been discontinued. The nurse had told the patient she shouldn't smoke for a couple of hours so the room would clear out, that she should take a shower because her clothes and hair were saturated with oxygen. This patient was too rambunctious and decided to light a cigarette. Poof, and her hair was all gone. When we walked into the room the patient was sitting there, totally bald, a black cigarette in her mouth."

When the topping-out of the new hospital took place on April 24, 1974, Sister Stella Louise reminded the audience: "In 1967 when we first began a long-range plan of healthcare in this community, there were some who expected us to move from the city—to flee the neighborhood we had so many years been part of and dedicated to.

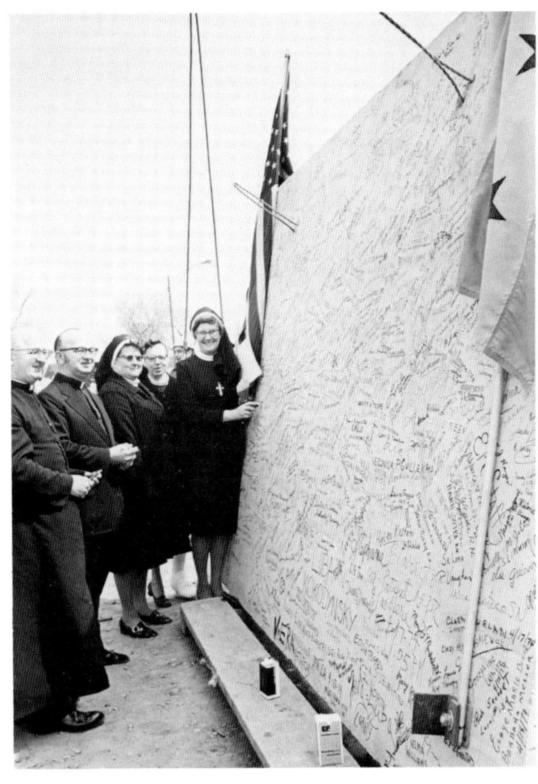

The Rev. Walter Krempa, chaplain of Saint Mary's; the Rev. Norbert Wachowiak, pastor of St. Helen's Church; Sister Rosemary; Sister Michaeline; and Sister Stella Louise admire over one thousand employee signatures on the last cement slab of the new hospital center.

We did not leave; we did not flee. This building being topped out today should be proof enough that we will stay and fulfill the pledge our Sisters made many years before."

In the 1973 annual report, Sister Stella Louise wrote a statement reminiscent of a previous time in the history of the Congregation: "We strained to fulfill our community health obligations in the outmoded facility in which we are housed."

The School of Nursing

In 1894 the idea of Sisters becoming nurses, of healing the body and ministering to the spirit, was entirely incompatible with popular social concepts. But shortly after the establishment of Saint Mary of Nazareth Hospital, the idea found an advocate in Dr. F.J. Laibe. On his visits to Mother Lauretta at the convent, he met Sister Mary Callista Konopacka, then a young religious. Believing she would make a good nurse, he undertook her instruction himself.

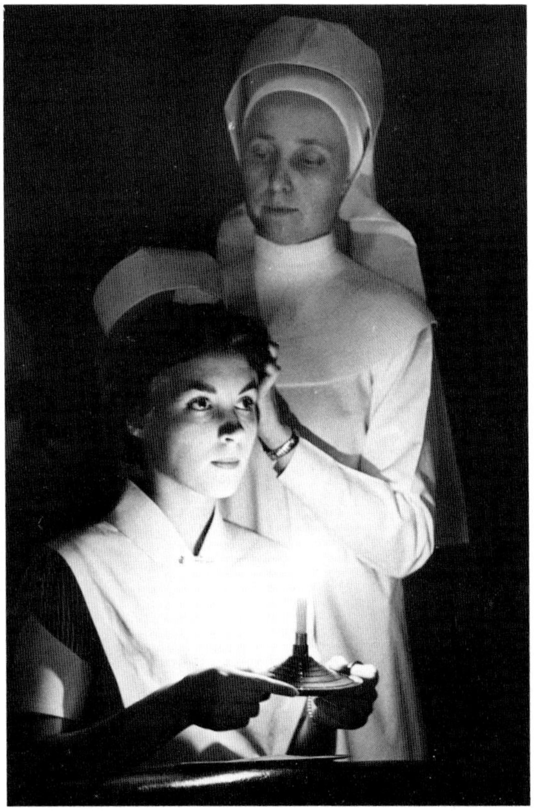

Sister Amata Sweeney capping a nurse (photo courtesy of the *Chicago Tribune*)

Dr. Albert Ochsner, appointed chief of the medical staff in 1896, enjoyed a highly respected reputation well beyond the limits of the hospital. He and the other doctors saw an urgent need for trained nurses in a hospital that was rapidly expanding and had a continuous increase in admissions. Dr. Ochsner told Mother Lauretta that the Sisters should have professional training and a nursing school should be established.

Mother Lauretta agreed. The Sisters, already nursing the sick to the best of their abilities, also had to help maintain the general upkeep of the institution. Early in 1900, through the efforts of Dr. Ochsner, she visited Sister Camilla, the Superior of St. Joseph's Hospital, to ask about acquiring a graduate nurse. Mother Lauretta was looking for someone who could assume responsibility as superintendent of nurses and had the skills to establish a curriculum for training nurses.

Theresa Smith, RN, was recruited and became the first director of nursing. With no set standards for schools of nursing in 1900, each hospital operated according to its own needs. Smith outlined the initial curriculum and successfully interested several young women in nursing careers. The School of Nursing thus became the hospital's first educational element, just six years after its founding.

In 1903 the school graduated its first class of seven nurses: one Sister and six lay women. In June of the same year, the school was incorporated under the laws of the State of Illinois.

The Alumnae Association was founded in 1911. The following year, the school was accredited by the State of Illinois. The first male nurse graduated in 1912. Accreditation by the National League for Nursing was conferred in 1952.

More space, more knowledge

Increased patient admissions were making the fifth floor of the hospital crowded. The student nurses resided there along with obstetrical patients. Plans for a separate residence for student nurses were begun in 1910 that finally saw fruition four years later.

In 1914 large additions were built at the north and south ends of the hospital. The nurses received a separate residence and school. Housing for interns and Sisters was expanded and space was added for private patient rooms, an enlarged laundry, a kitchen and a laboratory.

While the National League of Nursing Education endorsed the standards of the school and its curriculum, Mother Isabella—superintendent from 1925 to 1931—saw the need to raise academic standards. In 1928, high school graduation was instituted as a prerequisite for all applicants, although it was not compulsory in Illinois until 1937. In the late 1920s, a close relationship with De Paul University was developed. The school secured its affiliation with the university in 1931 through a contractual agreement with Dr. Joseph A. Tobin, director of the Department of Nursing. From that time on, non-nursing courses within the program of studies could be applied toward a bachelor of science degree in nursing.

Events of note

A follow-up study illustrated some interesting facts about some early graduates:

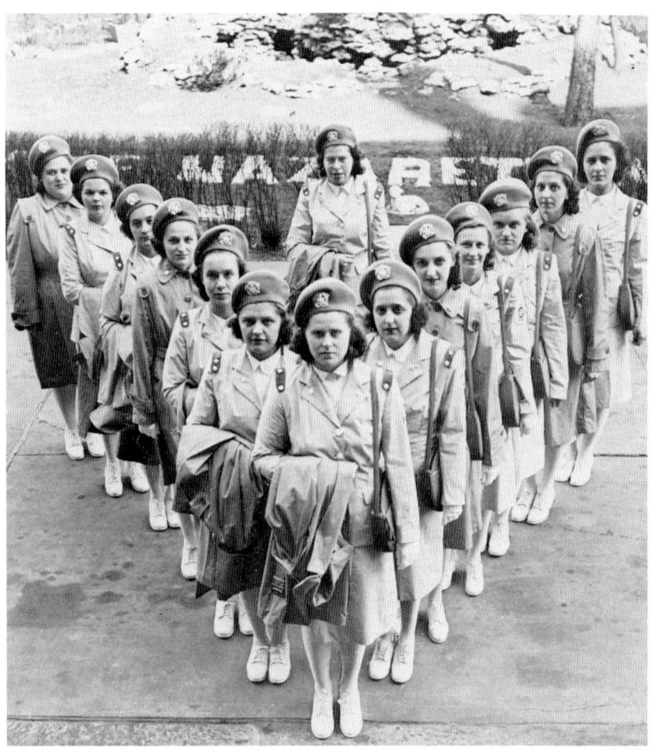

The Nursing Cadet Corps was a government program that paid tuition for nursing students in exchange for service in the Armed Forces, if needed, 1943.

Lieutenant Carolyn Little, class of 1903, was decorated by King George V at Buckingham Palace for distinguished service at the U.S. Base Hospital No. 11 at Nantes, France.

Helen Walderback, class of 1908, spent 25 years as director of nursing for St. Anne's Hospital School of Nursing.

Emily Skorupa, class of 1912, served with the American Red Cross in Poland during World War I. She later became director of the Poznan School of Nursing and translated the book *Home Hygiene and Care of the Sick* by Jane Delano into the Polish language for student distribution.

Mary L. Laibe, class of 1912, was superintendent of nurses at the Municipal Tuberculosis Sanitarium, a suburban Chicago hospital, and the Barrington Rest Home. She also taught home hygiene and home care of the sick for the American Red Cross.

Josephine Heerey, class of 1914, gave nursing care to underprivileged and undernourished children in her home.

Marie Czwalinski, class of 1926, was orthopedic nursing consultant at the University of Illinois, Division of Services for Crippled Children.

Ann Batts, class of 1930, served on the board of the first nurses' association and was district representative on the Joint Committee of the Women's Court and Detention Home.

A pre-entrance test was required for admission beginning in 1947, and a 44-hour week (including classes) was established. There was ongoing evaluation of the program of studies and affiliations in clinical experience with the Municipal Tuberculosis Sanitarium of Chicago, Illinois State School of Psychiatric Nursing and United States Nurse Cadet Corps Program. Throughout the years, school directors Sisters Therese Netzel, Altissima Wicklas and Amata Sweeney were instrumental in initiating and maintaining standards of education in keeping with the societal health needs and nursing educational trends.

Sister Amata left in 1965 to become administrator of Holy Family Hospital in Des Plaines, Illinois. Later she would serve a term on the General Council in Rome, Italy. Currently she is a governing board member.

Sister Mary Antonia Klausner, RN, MSN, was appointed director of the School of Nursing in August 1965. She held that position for 21 years, until the school closed. Now the director of Organization Standards and Education, Sister Antonia recently spoke about the school:

"In June of 1965, new Illinois State nursing legislation passed, permitting professional nursing programs to have educational plans of not less than two years." To meet growing challenges in

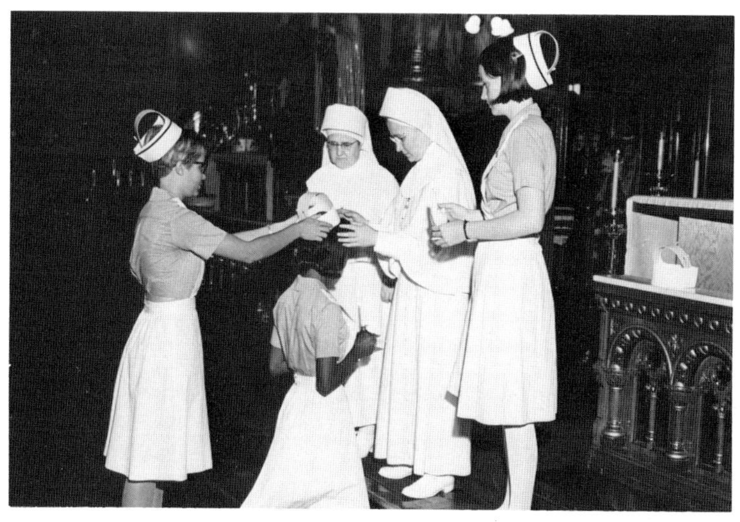

Sisters Agnes (left) and Antonia conduct the nursing school capping ceremony.

nursing education, the School of Nursing concluded its three-year program and inaugurated the two-year program in 1966. In 1968 the school graduated its last three-year program students (47) and its first two-year program students (59) for a total of 106 graduates, the largest graduating class in the school's history. "This new program," said Sister Antonia, "offered the same basic elements as were under the school's previous three-year plan."

In 1973, under provisions of the Health Services Education Grants Act, the school received over $59,000 in funds from the Illinois Board of Higher Education to establish a learning resources center. Computerized learning was implemented at this time.

Everyone worked hard

The nurses had a demanding schedule, with the newly revised program of studies. Sister Antonia had said she was "certain that by developing quality courses of shorter duration, we can graduate more nurses, while still maintaining high education standards." Administration and faculty were committed to sound education, and believed that "to teach is to touch a life forever."

Armella Bernacki, now Public Relations department secretary, worked in the school for 11 years. "I helped market the school, recruiting high school seniors in Chicago and the suburbs for career days; took care of the applications; set up interviews and testing dates; prepared letters of acceptance and rejection; maintained the files and took care of the grades and transcripts; typed the tests and catalog and ran them off on a ditto machine; prepared program books; did administrative secretarial work, and generally took care of the office for Sister."

Connie Drogos, RN, Human Resources Development, was a student during the late 1960s. "The rules were very strict. We couldn't enter or leave the school in anything but a skirt or dress. I remember leaving the building with my shorts or slacks under my skirt, then going around the corner and taking off my skirt! And we weren't allowed to wear any earrings or colored nail polish."

There were moments when levity

erupted spontaneously. Sister Kathleen, now assistant administrator, Continuing Care, recalls: "I was an instructor in the School of Nursing off and on for many years. Saint Mary's prepared hundreds of really good nurses. It's neat to see some of them who are still here who were my students—very competent and caring people. One of my favorite stories happened to a newly graduated nurse working night shift while we were still in the old building. She had this patient who was moaning. The lady—her name was Anna—absolutely would not stop moaning. She said over and over again, `Oh, God ... oh, God!' Everything possible had been done to relieve her pain and distress. On and on it went. She kept moaning: `Oh God, oh, God.' She was keeping the whole place awake. Finally, the nurse got on the intercom and said, Anna, this is God. I want you to be quiet now and go to sleep.' And she did."

High marks

"The students really had a full life," says Sister Antonia. "It wasn't just nurses studying nursing; they had a lot of social activities to develop fully. In the nursing building, there were also schools of anesthesiology, radiology and medical technology. It was nice, because these students had other students to enjoy their life with, to learn and recreate together. The schools worked cooperatively; many students became friends, sometimes even married. The school was a very dynamic, living place. We were alive, and we wanted our people to be alive. There wasn't anything left undone to make the students better—spiritually, financially, and

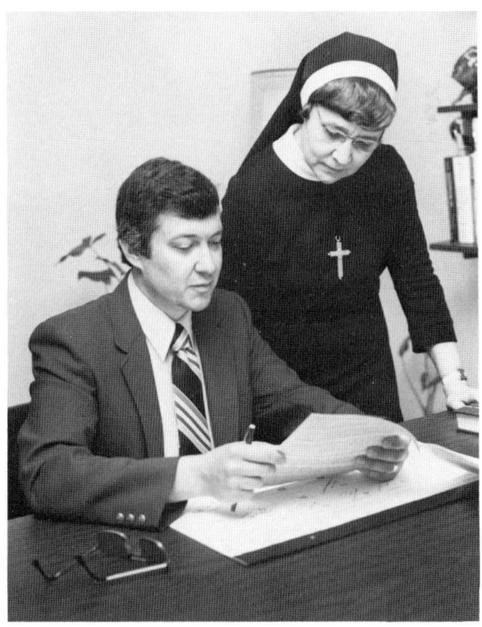

Sr. Antonia with former Director of Education Robert W. Matthews, PhD

educationally." Beginning in 1972, state and federal grants awarded to the school made it possible to implement innovations within the curriculum, provide for students' needs and enable dreams to come true for underprivileged students who might not otherwise be able to attend.

Sister Antonia produced a carefully preserved letter from an alumna: "I received the news of the School of Nursing closing with great sadness. Saint Mary's is a part of me and I owe my successful career to the excellent education I received at your and Sister Amata's hands. Because of the high moral, ethical and nursing standards you imprinted on me, I have enjoyed steady advancements into the position I hold today. In addition, I have been chapter president of a national nursing organization and have lectured at many hospitals and nursing homes and have published in two national journals. All this from a great school of nursing. Thank you for everything, Saint Mary's and you." Another alumna wrote, "Sister Antonia, your letter was very moving. I extend my best wishes to you. I have been and always will be proud of my school as it was the basis for my growth in military nursing. You are always with me wherever I am stationed in the United States or around the world."

In 1986 Sister Antonia summarized the school's achievements: "The School of Nursing has been in existence for 86 years. Since its founding, the school has added approximately 3,000 graduates to the ranks of those fully qualified for the noble and gentle art of nursing. Our graduates are meeting the health needs of people in the United States, in the European countries, and in the Third World. The School of Nursing has its own unique history, tradition, and pride. Excellence in education, dedication, `hands on' experience and preparation of nurses who give quality nursing care were always our goals. I am truly proud of the accomplishments of our graduates, their image, and continued education."

Resulting from a study by a Task Force on Education, Hospital Finances and Health Care Changes, the hospital closed the School of Nursing at the end of the 1985-86 academic year. The last graduation was held on June 21, 1986.

Sister Mary Agnes, now resource advisor for standards and quality of care for the medical-surgical areas, has held several posts spanning 52 years. She served in various positions, including convent superior and nursing school faculty member. From 1965 until 1975, she was director of nursing service. In 1975 she was elevated to assistant administrator for the Department of Nursing and remained in that position until 1984. During her tenure, she witnessed tremendous growth and was instrumental in creating a conducive environment for a progressive nursing department. She worked closely with the School of Nursing and supported faculty in all of their endeavors. Her concern was always the patient, therefore standards of care were developed and implemented. She spoke out clearly whenever the good of the patient was involved. 'I have made my own opinions known about certain things,' she said, 'often not too successfully. Like making visiting hours in ICU more liberal. You don't make standard rules. You allow visitors according to patient's needs. I once read in a book, `When the mother got well she said to her daughter, 'Instead of all the strangers around me I would have preferred that you sat there and held my hand. I would have gotten well much sooner."' I can be very proud that we have always been highly motivated and progressive to the extent that we've attempted to provide the best possible care to the patients with the newest techniques and ... been able to stand up to anybody and face them and say, `What we're doing here is the right thing at the right time.' '

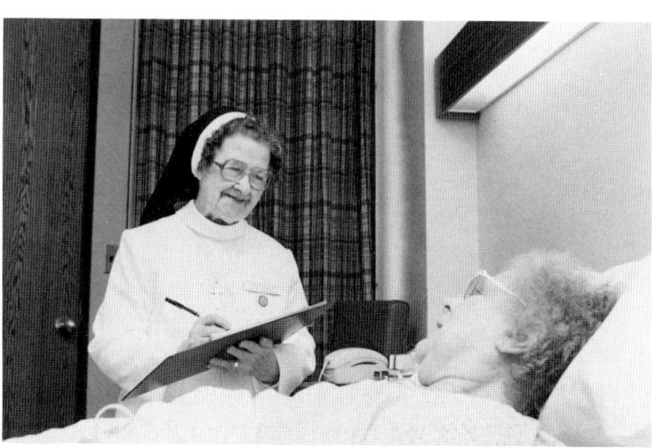

Sister Agnes makes her quality assessment rounds.

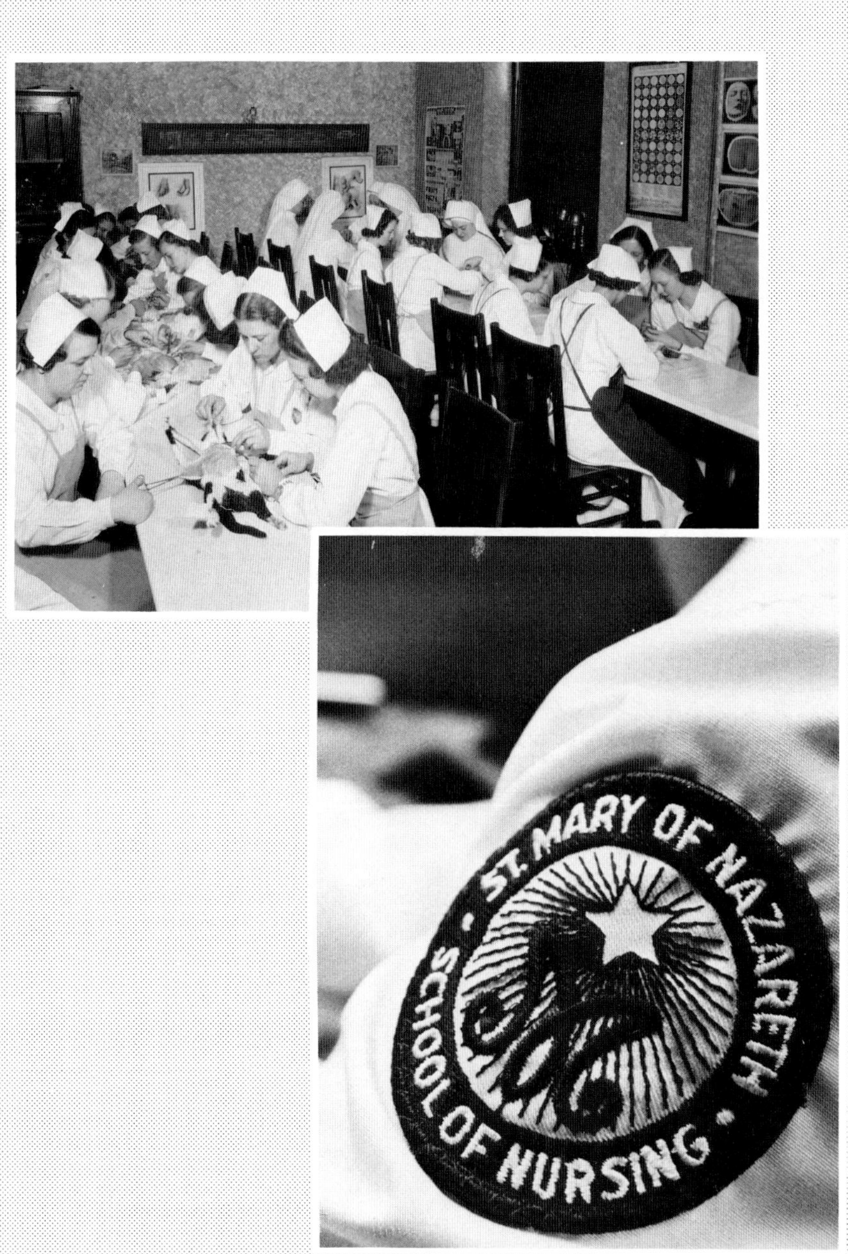
ST. MARY OF NAZARETH
SCHOOL OF NURSING

School of Nursing

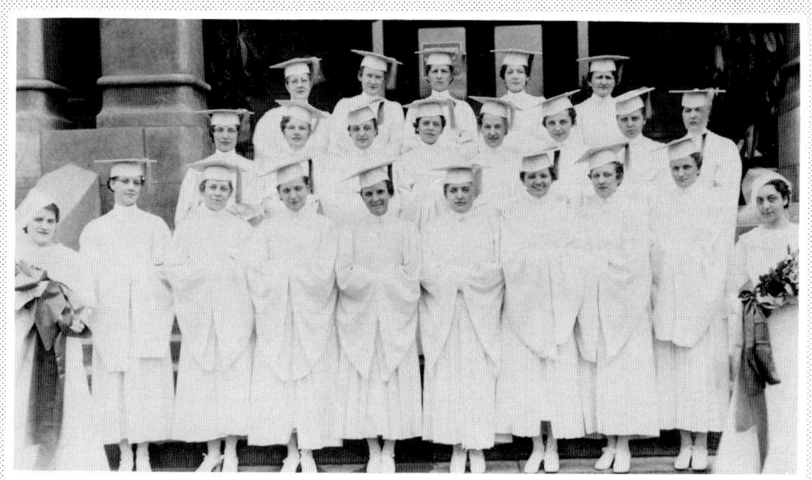

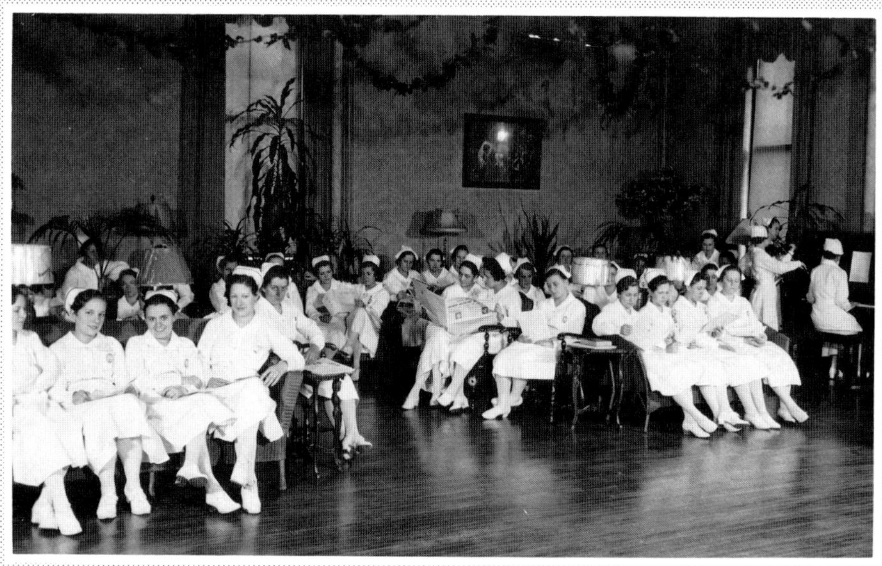

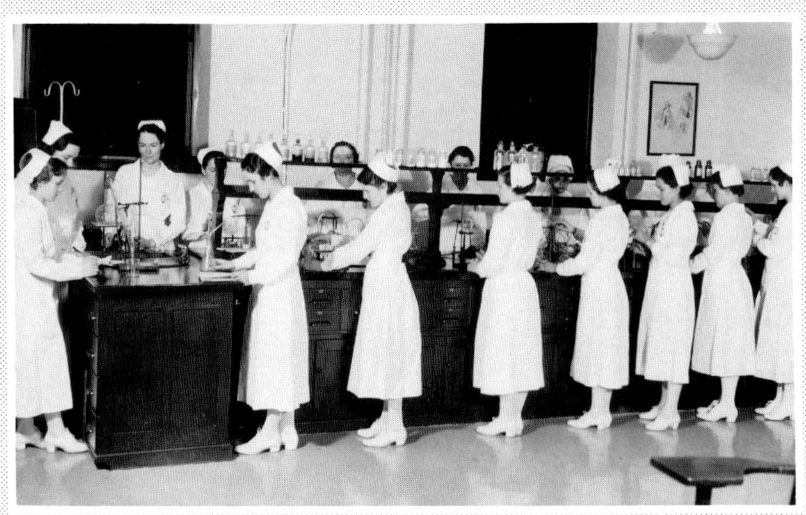

School of Nursing

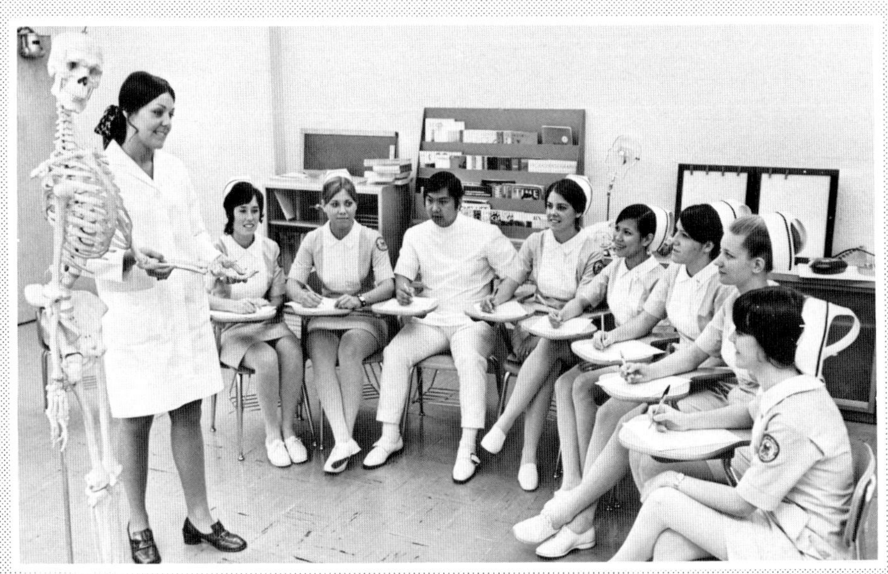

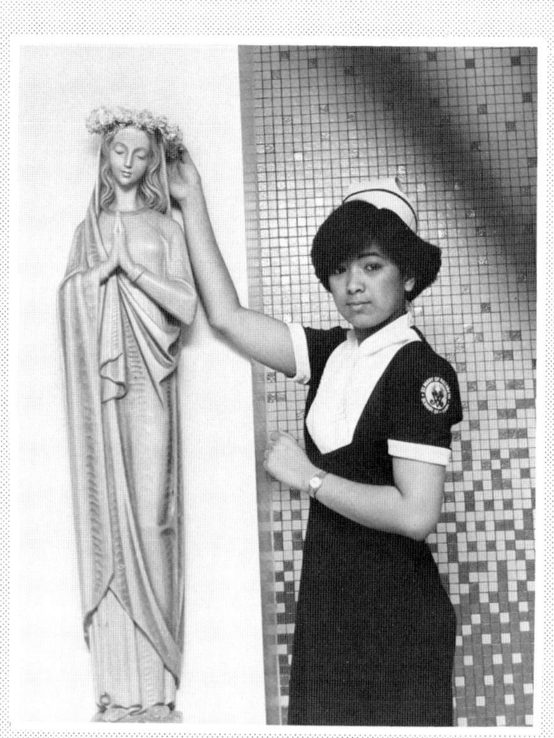

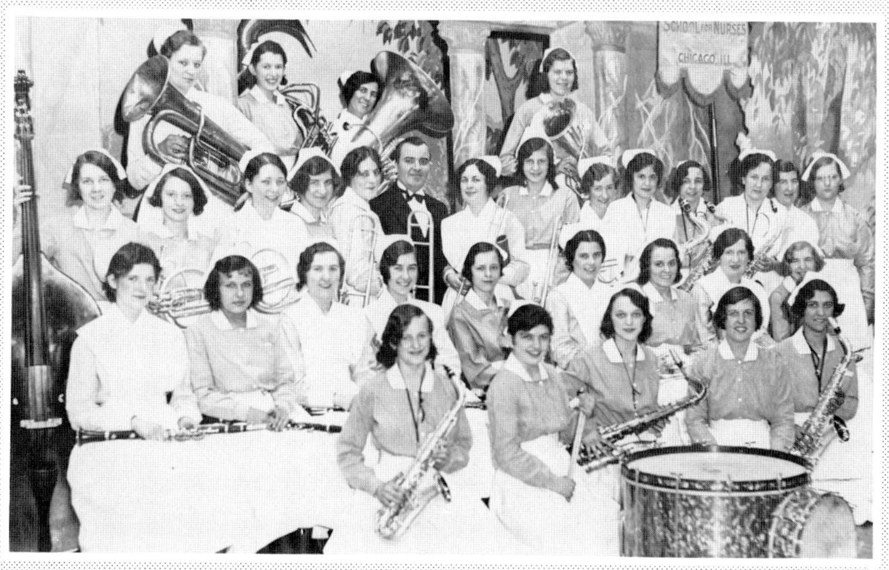
NURSES
CHICAGO

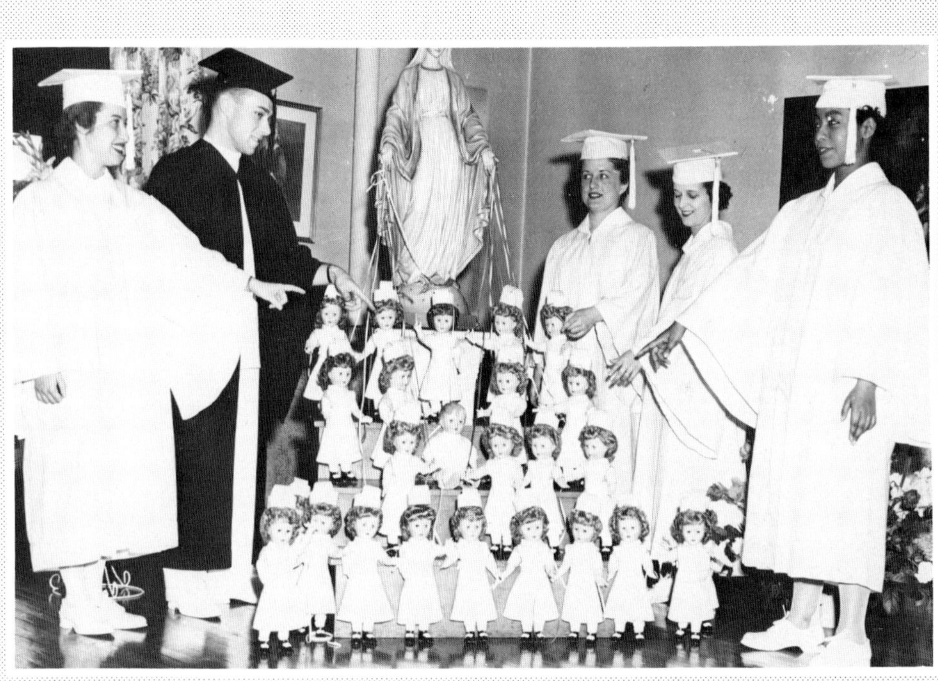

School of Nurse Anesthetists

Founded in 1934, the School of Nurse Anesthetists was in existence until the early 1960s. The primary purpose was to "educate registered nurses in the science and art of anesthesia—so that they will become efficient and skilled in administering the various methods of anesthetics intellectually and scientifically, in the spirit of kindness and charity."

In its preface, an early school catalog stated: "Anesthesia has been called a 'special type of nursing,' combining the

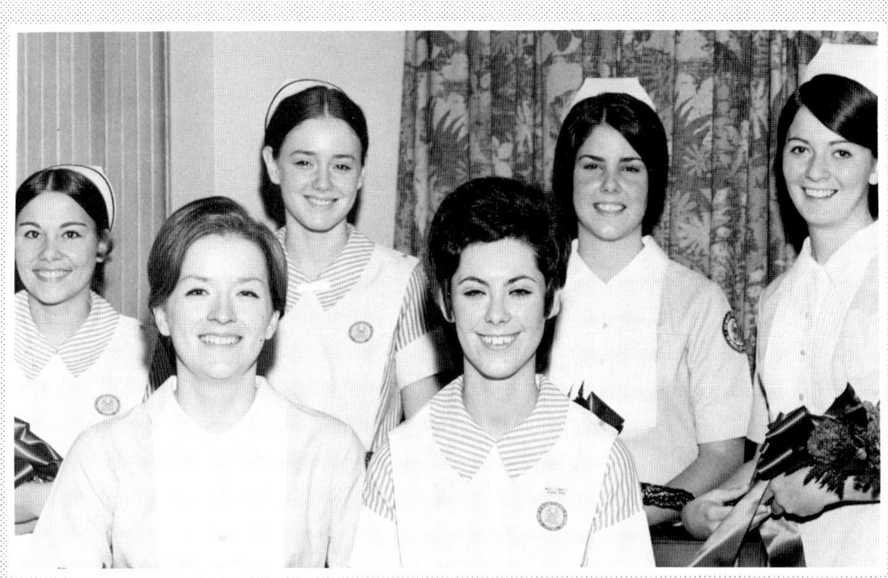

First year nursing school student Gail Coker (front row, left) is selected to represent students attending the 695 U.S. hospital nursing schools in the 1971 Rose Bowl Parade in Pasadena, California.

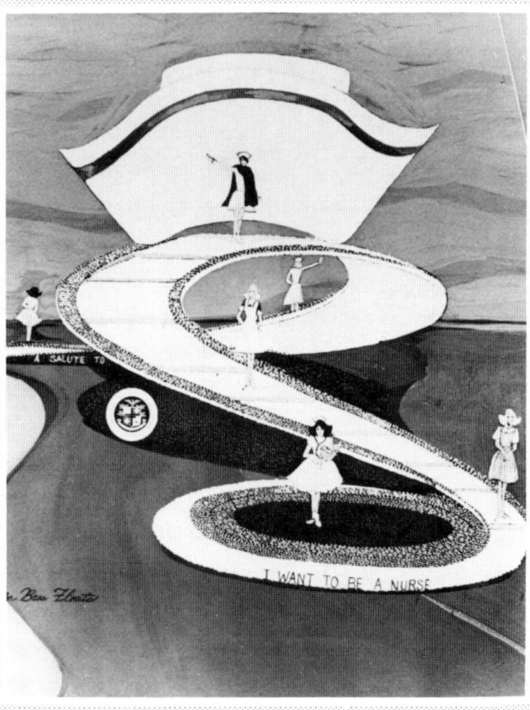

The 'I want to be a nurse' float was sponsored by the American Hospital Association.

gentle attentions and psychology of superior bedside nursing with the arts of technical nursing and the knowledge of advanced science. Much is required of the professional nurse who enters the field of anesthesia; but as an anesthetist she stands as an essential part of a surgical team. To qualify as an anesthetist, a nurse must be able at all times to command her mind, her hands, and her emotions."

The school offered an 18-month course in anesthesia, recognized by and conducted according to the requirements of the American Association of Nurse Anesthetists (AANA). Graduates were eligible to take the AANA qualifying membership exam and were also eligible for membership in the American Association of Inhalation Therapists.

Sisters Reginella and Domicile graduated from the school and then worked at the hospital.

School of Radiologic Technology

Saint Mary's established the X-Ray School in 1941, under the direction of Dr. Chester Challenger who held that post until his death in 1959. The curriculum was expanded to include nuclear medicine in 1962, and it became the School of Radiologic Technology. It was the first school of a private hospital in the Midwest to offer training in both radiologic technology and nuclear medicine. Dr. Donald C. Wharton was medical director from 1959 until the school closed.

The school was formally affiliated with Crane Junior College in 1965 so that it could offer an associate-degree program. The three-year course was the first such hospital-college cooperative educational arrangement in Illinois. The first students to complete this program received their degrees in July 1968.

William Plos, current director of Radiology, was the 1965 winner of the "Challenger Award," given to one senior of each graduating class for outstanding scholastic achievement.

After 40 years of operation, Saint Mary's School of Radiologic Technology graduated its last class on May 28, 1980.

School of Medical Technology

The School of Medical Technology was opened in 1950, directed by Sister Mary Wendeline, its first instructor.

A year-long program, the school was affiliated at various times with De Paul University, Mundelein College, Northern Illinois University and Illinois State University. It offered courses in hematology, chemistry, serology, bacteriology, blood bank, general analysis and histology. It provided the fourth year of work for a bachelor of science degree in medical technology. The school accepted students with three years of college or students from schools outside the United States who already had bachelor of science degrees.

Upon completing the program in medical technology, the student was eligible to take the national registry examination to be qualified and accredited by the American Society of Clinical Pathologists as a medical technologist. Recent technical directors of the school included Sister Celestine, Sister Ignatius and Rhonda (Hoskins) Konkel.

The words of Sister Stella Louise, herself a graduate of the School of Radiologic Sciences, could have applied as well to the schools of nursing and medical technology: "I am sorry to see the School of Radiologic Sciences close after 40 years of training students to be radiology technicians, but hard economic realities have forced the closing after years of rapidly increasing costs."

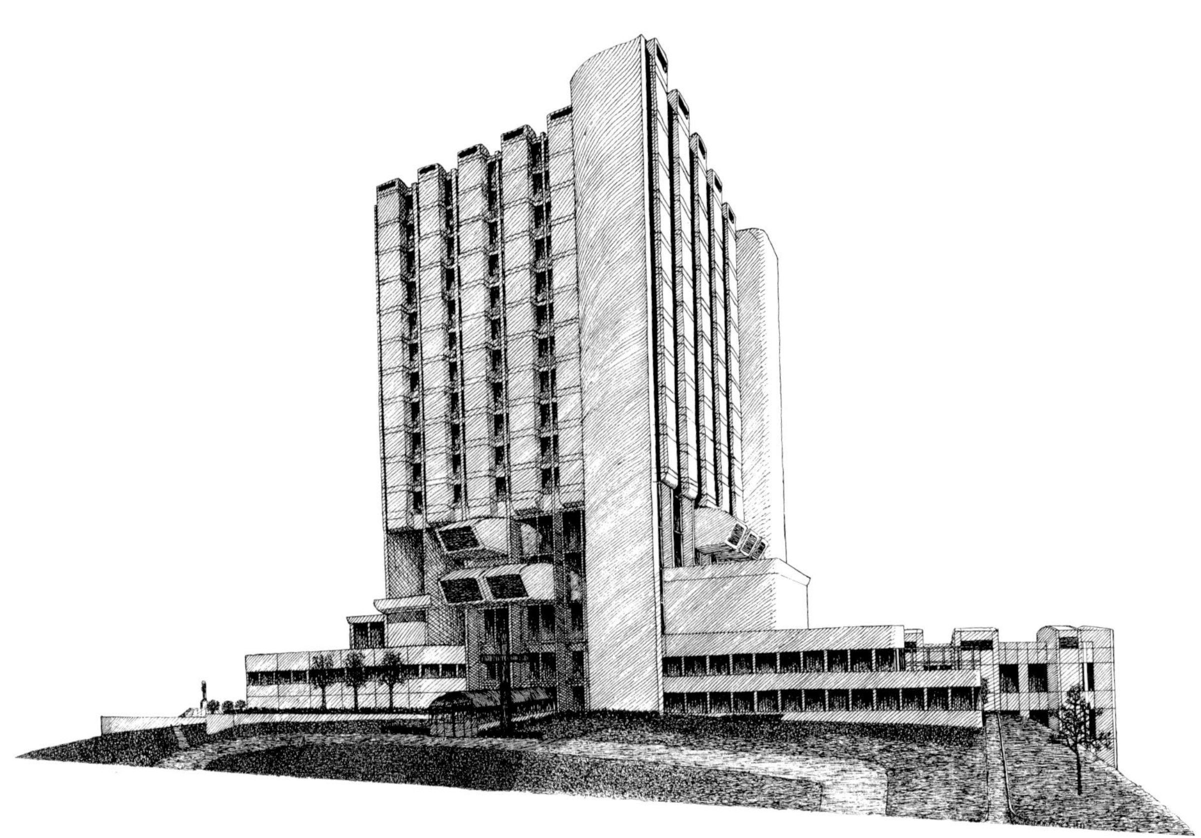

way the forms were positioned, after which the concrete was poured in place.

The unique Stations of the Cross were created by a local Jewish sculptress, Lee Schillereff. Sister Stella Louise gave the artist a book, *A Doctor Goes To Calvary*, and told her the figures had to be anatomically correct because the healthcare providers that would frequent the chapel would notice that. Doctors and nurses would know, for instance, that if nails were

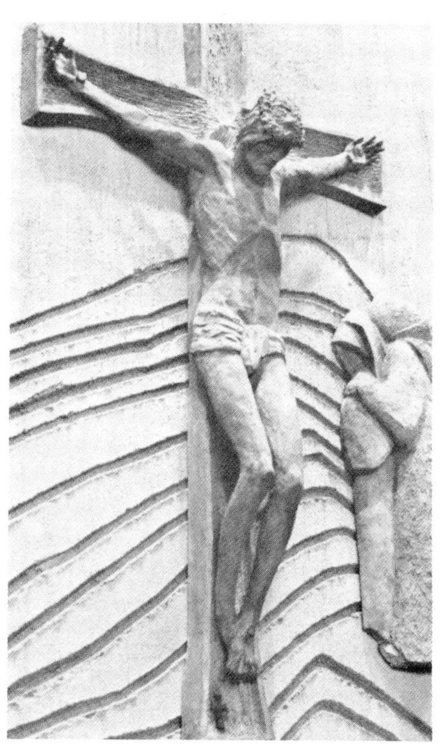

Station of the cross number twelve in the hospital chapel: Jesus crucified

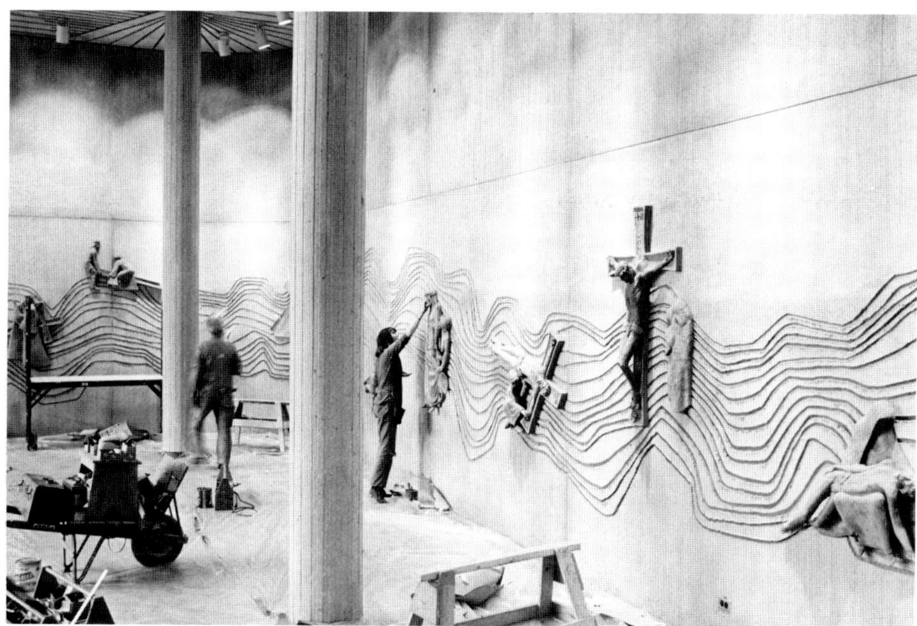

Artist Lee Schilleriff creating stations of the cross, December, 1974.

driven through Christ's hand they would tear through. Thus the sculptress placed the nails through the wrists. So that patients can relate better with the suffering Christ, all the stations are larger than in most chapels. The artist made lines in the wet cement between the Stations of the Cross to symbolize the winding path to Calvary. The theme of the altar tree and the path centers on the tabernacle.

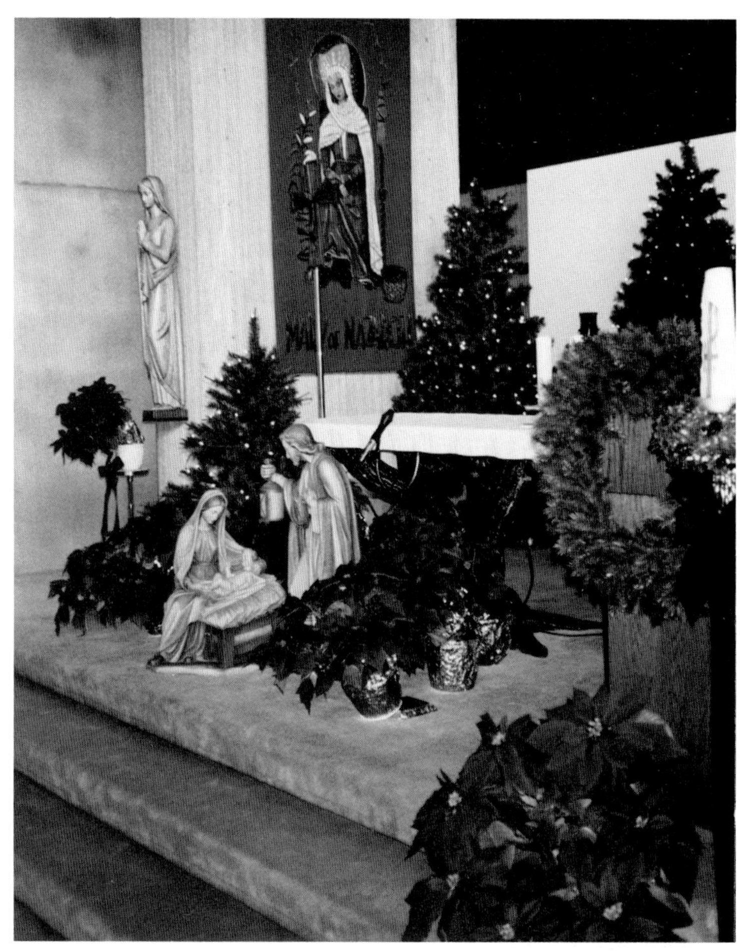

The hospital chapel at Christmas

The rustic-looking altar symbolizes the tree of life. The symmetry, texture and design of the sanctuary lend architectural and artistic unity of form and composition.

The chapel serves as the heart of the hospital community. Masses are offered daily for employees, medical staff and visitors, transmitted via closed-circuit TV to patient rooms. Liturgical celebrations are held throughout the year, including Holy Week services, St. Luke's Day (Patron Saint of Physicians), Dr. Martin Luther King Jr. prayer service, May crowning, Christmas (including midnight mass), holy days of obligation and feast days.

Father John Kobus gives a homily at Mass.

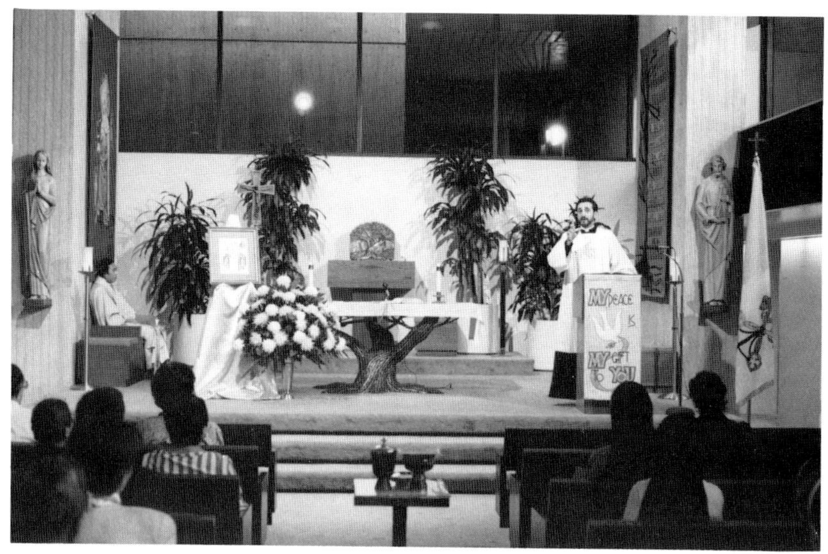

A special visit

On August 20, 1976, a delegation of the Episcopate of Poland headed by Karol Cardinal Wojtyla visited Saint Mary's. Mayor Richard J. Daley and John Cardinal Cody were present, as Saint Mary's was the official City of Chicago welcoming site. After a press conference, Cardinal Wojtyla and his 15 accompanying bishops toured the hospital. The Polish Cardinal was particularly impressed with the chapel. He knelt in the front pew, admiring the appearance of the altar and the sanctuary.

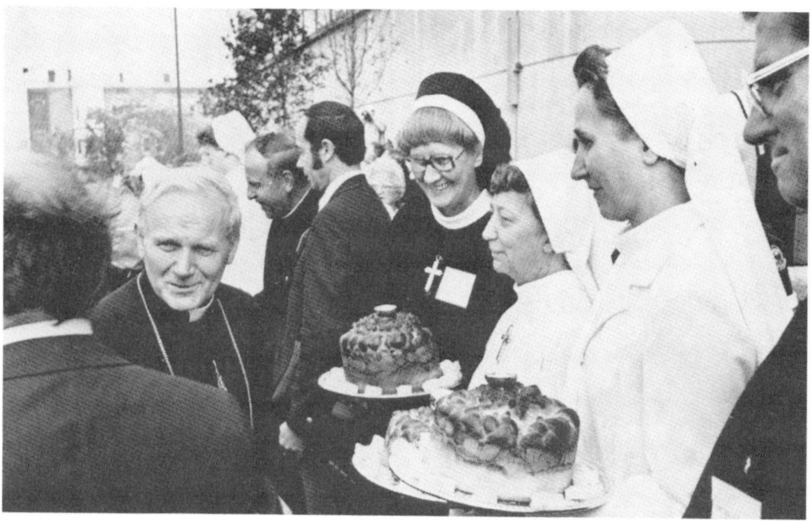

Touring U.S. cities in August, 1976, visiting bishops from Poland were treated to a traditional welcome of bread, symbolizing material sustenance, and salt, signifying spiritual sustenance. Kenneth Colby, Personnel Manager, baked the loaves. Offering the bread to Cardinal Wojtyla were, from left, Sister Stella Louise, Sister Gabrielle and Sister Patricia Ann.

Two years later, Cardinal Wojtyla was elected the Supreme Pontiff and took the name of Pope John Paul II. His election brought joy to the Sisters and staff. Steeped in a tradition of Polish heritage, Saint Mary's and the Congregation were especially proud and joyous over the election of the first Polish Pope in the history of the Catholic Church.

Symbols of reverence

In 1975 Marianne and Wayne Hamilton, hospital employees for a combined 25 years at that time, paid tribute to the concepts that had led to the founding of Saint Mary's and the United States by donating a flagpole to the hospital. This gesture memorialized the country's

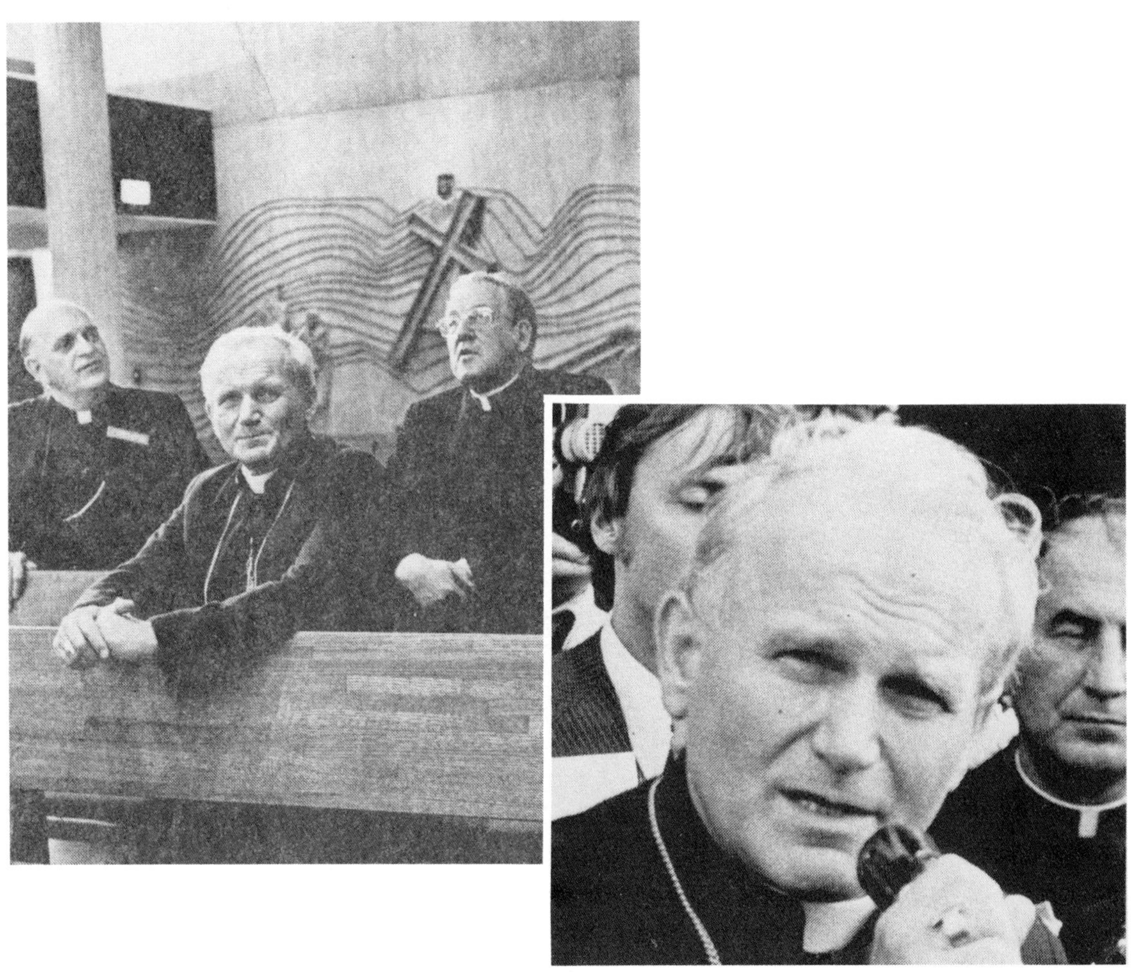

Bicentennial and was placed to honor Chester and Anne Koziol and Percy and Anne Hamilton, their parents.

The following year, a cross was erected near the main entrance. Twenty-eight feet high, with a span of 16 feet, the cross weighs 4,000 pounds and was manufactured from structural steel. It symbolizes the force behind the Sisters' mission: Catholic healthcare ministry.

Celebrating the building's first birthday on March 10, 1976, Sister Stella Louise planted a seven-foot pin oak tree on the front lawn. The oak, with its deep roots, was chosen as a symbol of the dedication of the Sisters of the Holy Family of Nazareth to the community.

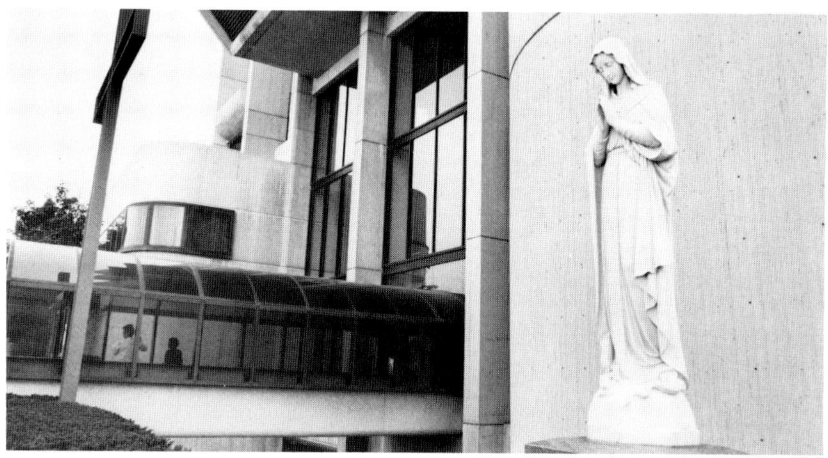

In 1976 the statue of the Blessed Virgin that had stood in front of the Leavitt Street hospital for 32 years was moved to the emergency parking circle. Later, when the helipad was built, it would return to the front of the new hospital. A gift from the Sisters of the Immaculate Conception Province in Torresdale, Pennsylvania, the statue was given in honor of Saint Mary's Golden Jubilee in 1944.

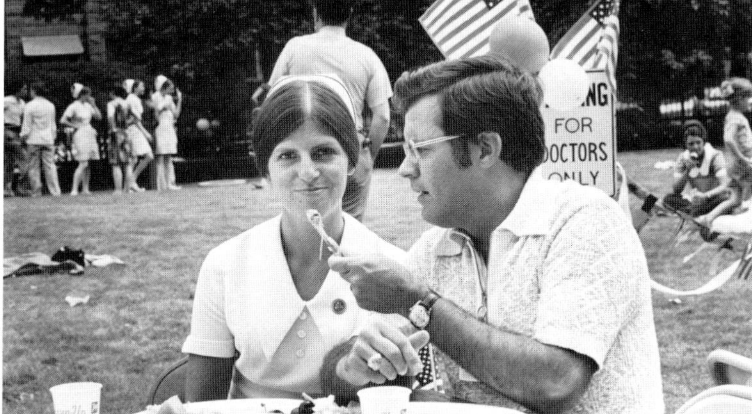

Newlyweds Marianne Koziol Hamilton, RN, Nursing Supervisor, and C. Wayne Hamilton, Assistant Administrator for Materials Management, enjoy the 1973 employee lawn party.

Memories of My Father's Place

I recall the day many years ago
My father planted four locust trees in a row.
Sitting on the bench of my memories
I watched his kind tending
Being present to his caring love.

At another time, in another place
I beheld my "Father's tree" in a masterpiece
Where the tree and artist met.
Again, sitting on the bench of my memories
Being present to his creative beauty.

In the midst of daily ministry, doing my Father's will
In the home of my Father, I hear the call, His house to rebuild
Ah, yes, in my Father's place
My Father's altar tree must be
Being present to His redeeming love.

Now in my Father's house
Sitting on the bench of my memories
I bring my own and others' broken bent branches
To be grafted and bonded with His own
Being present to His healing balm.

—Sister Stella Louise, CSFN

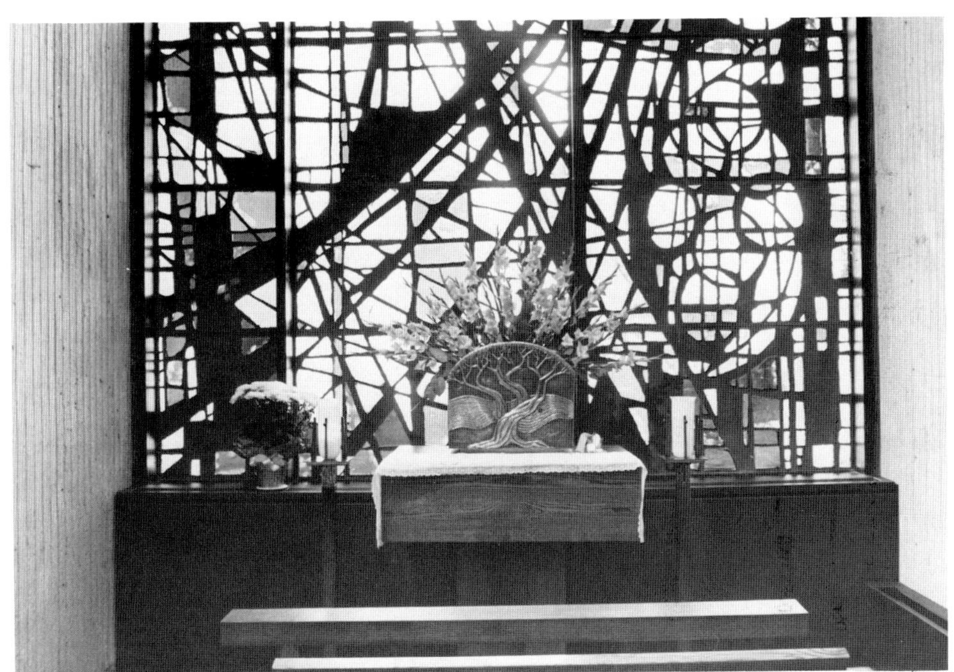

The Blessed Sacrament Tabernacle in the Meditation Chapel

Dr. Przypyszny has very strong connections to the original mission of the hospital and its Polish origins. His uncle served as a chaplain during the 1940s and 1950s. His mother, aunt and wife were all nurses here. His father was a surgeon and general practitioner on staff. Dr. Przypyszny considers his following in his father's profession as entirely logical. 'When my father died I just took over his practice.'

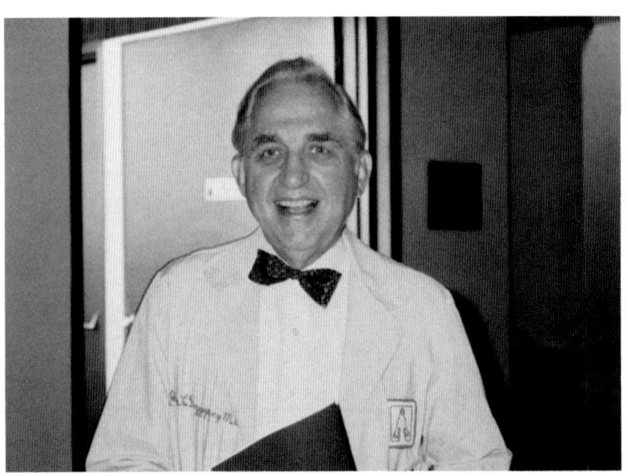

Dr. John C. Przypyszny MD, 1994 Medical Staff President and Utilization Review Medical Director

His typical day is quite full. Up by 5:30 a.m., at the hospital by 6:30, he takes care of utilization review—of which he is in charge—then makes rounds on patients. 'Patient load is lighter for me and for all doctors,' he reports. 'When I came here we had patients admitted for a couple of days just to find out what was going on. I don't have one-third the patient load I had before. Most surgery is ambulatory these days.' When it's brought to his attention that despite his reduced schedule he still puts in 12- to 13-hour days, he responds: 'Well, it's a routine. Everybody sets their routine.'

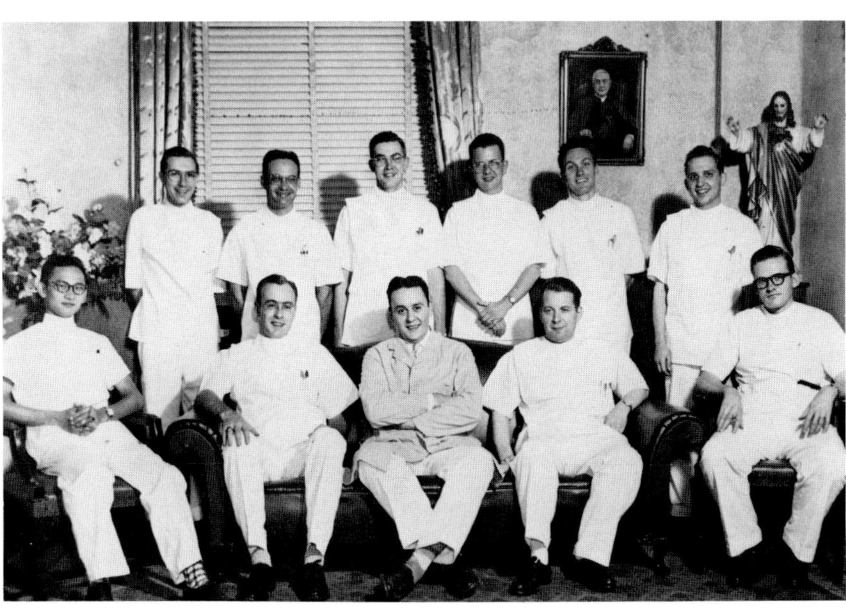

Dr. Przypyszny as a young intern (standing, far right)

Examples of leadership

Sister Mary Floriann, open heart nurse coordinator, offers a capsulized history of Saint Mary's cardiac care: "In 1967, Dr. Salvatore Motto, chief of Cardiology at that time, opened our first Intensive Coronary Care Unit, which was equipped to do continuous ECG monitoring. The invasive hemodynamic pressure monitoring was introduced in 1975 in the new building. The Cardiac Catheterization and Special Procedures Laboratory was completed in January 1976. The Open Heart Surgery Program was crystallized in 1978 and was the only alternative treatment for coronary disease in addition to the medical therapy. The breakthrough for another alternative treatment of coronary disease came in 1984 when Dr. John Monteverde performed the first percutaneous transluminal coronary angioplasty (PTCA).

The Cardiac Catheterization/Special Procedures Department opened in 1976, providing physicians with angiographic and hemodynamic information related to obstructive blood-vessel disease. In 1977, Saint Mary's was the first hospital to begin using a computerized electrocardiograph system, and also provided access to the system by several other hospitals. It was christened "Sammy" after Dr. Salvatore Motto.

The Heart Club was founded in 1978 through the efforts of Dr. Motto and Sister Floriann for the benefit and support of heart patients and others interested in learning more about heart health.

Radiology, with its array of radiography, computerized tomography (CT), nuclear medicine and radiation therapy equipment, is strategically located

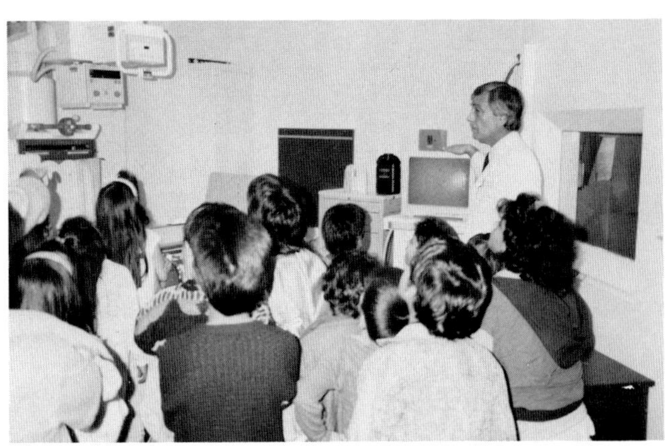

Director of Radiology Bill Plos demonstrates equipment for grammar school students during a hospital field trip.

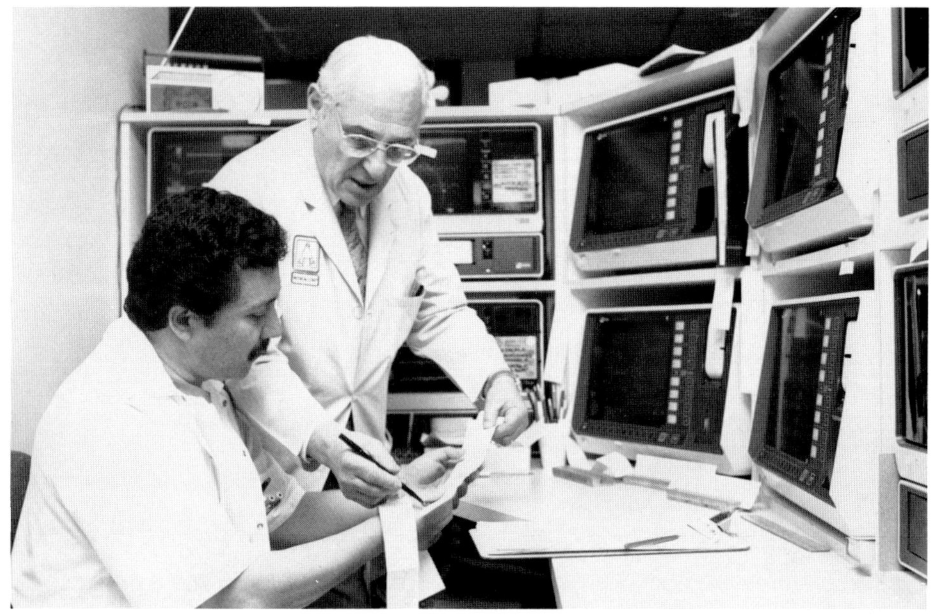

Cardiology Chairman Emeritus Salvatore A. Motto, MD, in addition to his many accomplishments as a physician, has always expanded the causes of the Sisters and the reputation of the hospital. Even though he is now retired from practice, he has not retired from Saint Mary's.

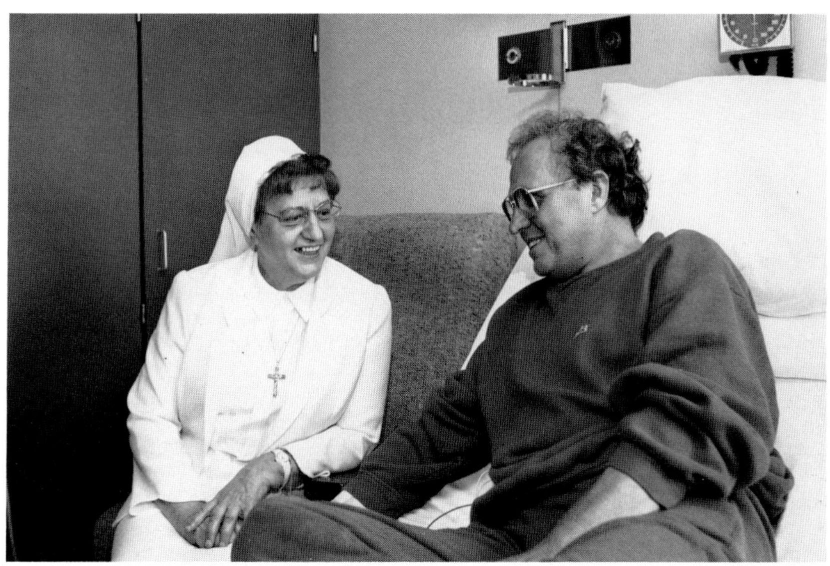

Sister Floriann with a cardiology patient

on the first floor to best serve the departments that need it. Magnetic resonance imaging (MRI) is located just outside the emergency room in a separate building. Bill Plos, RT, director of radiology, explains that the concept of radiology being located next to surgery, critical care and emergency is excellent. "All quick-response situations are in the same area."

Plos, married to Mary Ann Kroplewski, a radiology technologist he met at Saint Mary's in 1967, has about 60 employees under his direction. He says, "I've seen a lot of changes in the hospital—people and technology—but the patient has always been number one, always family-centered care."

In 1987, William V. Mollihan, MD, became only the third medical director of radiology in the hospital's history. He follows Donald C. Wharton, MD, who in 1959 succeeded founder Chester Challenger, MD.

Dr. Gerald Sunko directs radiation therapy. He has also served as an eucharistic minister to oncology patients. He came to the hospital in July 1976. He believes "Saint Mary of Nazareth Hospital Center strengthened themselves when they built the new hospital and founded the radiation therapy section." Dr. Sunko notes that, unlike some institutions, Saint Mary's has a high level of teamwork between the surgeons and therapists. "We have a lot of cooperation here and the patients are the beneficiary of that."

Values expressed

Two Saint Mary's publications have chronicled the comings and goings and activities of staff and employees: *Saint Mary's Life* and *Shibboleth*. Among their pages can be found some expressions of belief, as when Wayne Hamilton summarized the charism and mission of the Congregation on preserving Christian family life:

"The Respect Life Program continually stresses the inherent sanctity and dignity of each and every human being from conception until natural death. The program encourages those things which sustain, nourish or provide for the proper enjoyment of life, while opposing those that destroy or diminish human life. In 1978 and 1979 the Respect Life theme centers on the family. This focus is important because it's in the family that life originates, and where life is nurtured and sustained. It is in the family, too, that each person comes to know and love himself or herself and begins to realize his or her responsibilities to others. All of us in our own experiences here in our health care apostolate have become aware of the need to help families survive and flourish in an atmosphere enriched by faith and Christian values. We've enhanced several programs to promote the Sisters of the Holy Family of Nazareth's dedication to these principles."

An article titled "Perspective: Employee and Patient Loyalty" stated: "Commendable loyalty is a feature of this hospital that even the casual visitor can notice, and it may be that this underlying characteristic draws patients to Saint Mary's where the atmosphere is friendly and congenial." Sister Stella Louise says, "We think this loyalty is due to the feeling of spiritual camaraderie and Christian compassion emanated throughout the hospital by staff members. Employees not only care for their patients, but they care for their co-workers."

Former Volunteer Supervisor Dee Ward adds: "People really do care about each other here, and treat each other with respect and friendliness regardless of ethnic origin. Even though I am not a Catholic, I appreciate the religious atmosphere found here. It's good to be aware of other types of religion and I like the idea that special liturgical services are provided for patients and staff."

In the 1978 *Annual Report*, Sister Stella Louise wrote: "We can view 1978 as another year of vibrant proof that each caring person here truly is part of a spiritual entity that evolves into something more than quality care for the patient and a family-like closeness. Taken together, the people of Saint Mary's working for and with patients become a blessing, a gift from God, a mystery of mercy."

"During 1985 our Governing Board responded to major questions no one would have thought to ask 10 years ago. Do we have the financial resources, the personnel and the will to maintain our identity as a Catholic institution in the face of changing values and attitudes about the sick, disabled and poor? Does fiscal survival demand too many compromises

CRISIS! Saint Mary's Responds

It happened on a day the hospital celebrates each year as Founder's Day. The Annual Employee Recognition Dinner was scheduled for that evening, honoring those employees with service anniversaries.

On May 6, 1981, at approximately 2:30 p.m., thirteen injured children were rushed to the Emergency Department after they were struck by a car that went out of control near Chopin School, 2400 West Rice Street. By 3:00 p.m., 18 children had been brought to the hospital. "Since the children started coming in at shift change time, we had enough staff in all areas to handle the increased patient load, so it was not necessary to put the disaster plan into effect. Response to the crisis was extremely efficient. The situation was well controlled and calm, and the entire hospital staff functioned in an exemplary manner," Barry Millman, then vice president of operations, said.

Phyllis Pavese, Public Relations, says she will never forget that day. "About 2:30 p.m. we received a call from Channel 5 News, who monitors the police radio band. The reporter said they heard that several children had been injured, possibly in a school bus accident. Since our offices were then in the Education Building, I headed over to the hospital to get the information we needed directly from the Emergency Department. The wailing of sirens—not one, but lots of them—greeted me as I walked outside, and a chill went through me. As I arrived in ER, the first injured children were being brought in."

Patients were cared for in both the Emergency and Outpatient Departments. Other areas were called upon to provide additional staff. Families of the patients were directed to the Emergency and Radiology waiting rooms, where Pastoral Care and Social Work staff provided counseling.

Newspaper, radio and television reporters arrived at the hospital by 3:00 p.m. They were allowed to set up their cameras outside the Emergency Room, near Security's communications desk. Public Relations was responsible for the control of the news media and for giving them patient information.

continued

CRISIS! Saint Mary's Responds

"Normally in a situation of this sort," Pavese continued, "under the city's disaster plan, injured victims are dispersed by the Chicago Fire Department to various hospitals to avoid overloading. However, there were two policemen at the school who were sitting in their squad car when the accident occurred. They yelled into their radio to get any available units to the school and ran to help the injured kids. Policemen from all over the area came and drove nearly all the injured children to Saint Mary's in their vehicles."

Mayor Jane Byrne, Police Superintendent Richard Brzeczek, Department of Human Services Commissioner Lenore Cartwright, Chicago School Superintendent Ruth Love, and workers from the Department of Human Resources came to the hospital to offer assistance. The departments of Emergency, Outpatient, Social Work, Pastoral Care, Security, Public Relations, Radiology, Laboratory, Admitting, Respiratory Therapy, ICU, Surgery, Nursing, Mental Health, Anesthesia and Supply, Processing and Distribution (SPD) worked together to manage the crisis. Volunteer interpreters (many of the patients' families spoke only Spanish) came from several departments to help.

One child died soon after being brought to the hospital. Nine children were released on May 6, three more left the next day, and six had slightly longer stays. One of the most severely injured children had to be transferred to another hospital for a CT scan, as Saint Mary's did not have a scanner at that time. Upon learning that, Mayor Byrne and Police Superintendent Brzeczek (a former employee) vowed to help Saint Mary's acquire one, as they had been so impressed with how the staff handled the disaster. Brzeczek agreed to be the 1982 Recognition Award honoree, with the funds going toward acquiring a CT scanner. Mayor Byrne came to the 1981 Medical Staff Benefit to thank the doctors for donating to the same cause. Employees donated funds from their annual drive as well.

"I'm proud of the quick, efficient and skillful response of our staff, especially on the short notice they received. Two hours after the first children arrived, the Emergency and Outpatient departments were cleared, and the nine children who were admitted were being cared for in ICU, Surgery and Pediatrics. I thank all those who worked hard to save their lives," Sister Stella Louise said.

with the essential spirit of a Catholic healing ministry? Shall we allow our ethic of service to be replaced by an ethic of competition? How will we preserve our healthcare mission and maintain a viable healthcare ministry when the trend toward commercialized healthcare is advancing so rapidly?

"For several years our Governing Board faced the challenges that these questions pose. In 1985 we began charting a future course that will lead, not merely to Saint Mary's survival, but to re-establishment of a ministry that remains faithful to the hospital's essential mission as an exemplar of Christian healing."
—Sister Stella Louise, 1985 Annual Report

The government enters the picture

Major new financial worries and woes among America's healthcare providers and their patients began with the addition of Title XVIII, Medicare, to the Social Security Act in 1965, followed very shortly by Title XIX, Medicaid. The introduction of these programs and those to follow, such as the Prospective Payment System in 1984, have caused dramatic changes in the healthcare environment. Since 1965, government funding has contributed to Saint Mary's financial concerns. As early as the summer of 1978, an article in *Saint Mary's Life* was titled "Can the Catholic Hospital Survive with Increased Government Funding?" It pointed out that under national health insurance, federal and state aid may give government officials the right to dictate how these funds should be used: "The answer lies in a balance between public accountability and the Church's legitimate interest in maintaining autonomy and authority over its institutions."

Thomas O. Meirink, executive vice president, Operations, recalls that in the mid-1980s, both the state and federal governments initiated efforts to reduce the ever-escalating costs of healthcare through the Illinois Competitive Access and Reimbursement Equity (ICARE) Program and the Medicare Prospective Payment System (PPS). The clear intent of the government was to ratchet down the reimbursement for both physicians and hospitals to shrink widening budget

Statement of Philosophy

Saint Mary of Nazareth Hospital Center, as a Catholic healthcare facility, is a community of men and women whose efforts are directed to the care, comfort and healing of the sick and injured. This direction flows from the Gospel of Jesus Christ, who in His Life touched the brokenness of body, mind and spirit, and from the spiritual legacy of the Sisters of the Congregation of the Holy Family of Nazareth, called by Christ to cooperate with Him and His Church in extending the Kingdom of God's love by imitating Jesus, Mary and Joseph. The healing ministry of this hospital is rooted in the belief that human life, at every moment and in all conditions, is sacred and leads toward a union with God. Thus, all aspects of human existence, even death itself, are special and deserving of respect. The hospital conceives of healing as an act more fundamental than the clinical practice of medicine, and, through the grace of Christ's love, each member of the institution cooperates with Christ in bringing healing to all who enter its doors. Thus, through mutual compassionate service, each member of the hospital community can bear witness to the Kingdom of God's love.

The hospital's Christian healing ministry combines modern techniques of medical treatment and patient care with deep and genuine concern for the total welfare of each patient and his or her family. A competently trained medical and hospital staff, rooted in the love of God and strengthened through prayer, participates in this healing ministry by rendering a full range of medical, social, psychological and pastoral care services. As a Catholic institution, the hospital promotes the Church's teaching concerning medical ethics, social justice and reverence for life, and actively joins with all other institutions committed to those teachings. The hospital fosters appropriate education for physicians, healthcare professionals and all other hospital staff, so as to affirm the concept of a Christian ministry of healing.

The hospital, through its ministry of Christian healing and teaching, strives to address the healthcare needs of its patients and staff and community as well. In this way, the hospital is a healing agent and a witness to the Kingdom of God among His people in the here and now, and points to the fullness of that Kingdom in which we will discover His great love for our greater joy and heavenly peace.

deficits. Both ICARE and PPS and their successive programs would prove to have profound and long-lasting effects on Saint Mary's and all hospitals with large numbers of Medicare and public-aid-sponsored patients.

Meirink recounts how the hospital reacted by significantly reducing operating expenses, re-examining its organization and corporate culture, and diversifying its services to generate additional revenue to support its primary mission of healthcare. Diversification included the establishment and incorporation of STaMANA (a for-profit corporation), purchase and expansion of a commercial print shop, and development of the MedStop urgent-care facility. An occupational health service—JOBMED—and an audiology service were established. The emergency department improved nursing and physician skills so that Saint Mary's was designated an associate hospital in the state's emergency medical services system. A building on the northwest side of Chicago was purchased to accommodate a new home health agency. The hospital became a founding member of Chicago Metro Care, a health maintenance organization (HMO). The family practice residency program became a provider site for Blue Cross/Blue Shield's HMO Illinois. And MedStar—an air ambulance helicopter program—was launched.

Sister Stella Louise, responding to economic pressures in a 1986 *Saint Mary's Life* editorial, summed up by saying: "Let's replace worry with care!"

An aerial exploration

October 15, 1984, was the first day of operation for MedStar, an aeromedical service for emergency transport. The blue and white Long-Ranger II helicopter was staffed by a flight nurse trained as a critical care nursing specialist, a flight paramedic, a pilot trained in emergency transport and, when necessary, a flight physician. The helicopter and crew supplemented ambulances when long distance, traffic congestion or bad weather hampered a patient's chance for survival.

Aeromedical service has the potential to take advantage of the "golden hour," those first important minutes after a serious injury that can make the difference between life and death for a patient.

Construction of the helipad began the same month. For a while, MedStar flights landed in the open field directly north of the hospital. The service was in operation for about two years.

Celebration and self-appraisal

During 1984, celebrations were held throughout the year, marking Saint Mary's 90th anniversary. "Ninety Years of Caring" was the theme, and a special logo was designed. Banners lined the

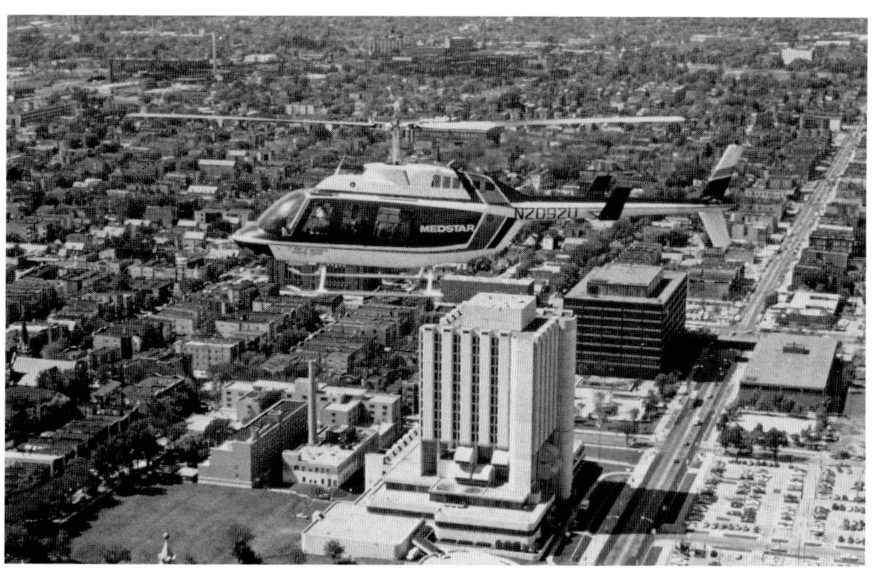

MedStar helicopter, 1986

surrounding streets, the annual report featured a festive birthday cake and streamers, and a "Gay 90s" lawn party was held with costumed employees and a horse-drawn carriage.

On the occasion of reaching ninety years, the hospital did a self-evaluation:

From memorabilia to museum

The Saint Mary of Nazareth Historical Museum—located on the third floor near the gift shop—was dedicated June 28, 1985, by Auxiliary Bishop Plácido Rodríguez, CMF. The opening coincided with the American centennial of the Sisters of the Holy Family of Nazareth.

The museum concept began with Wayne Hamilton, who had been saving memorabilia for years and had been affectionately dubbed 'Saint Mary's pack rat.' So many items had accumulated in his office that one day Sister Stella Louise commented, 'This place looks like a museum!' Her remark prompted Hamilton to ask Irene Allman of the Woman's Board to fund a museum project through their annual fashion show. They agreed, and the museum was fully funded by the board.

Project Director Phyllis Pavese, now director of Creative Services, worked with Curator Susan Phillips to design the museum and make the concept a reality. Phillips was hired through the 'Artists' Business Exchange Program' of the School of the Art Institute of Chicago, in order to provide a professionally curated exhibit. Donations were received from a wide variety of sources. Podiatrist Lee J. Kozie, DPM, donated an ENT (ear, nose and throat) chair and medical dressing cabinet that had been used by his father, Dr. Leon P. Kozakiewicz, who also had been on the hospital staff. Norm Millet, an architect from Perkins & Will (who designed the 1975 building) donated antique picture postcards depicting views of the hospital. The cards were found at a suburban antique show.

The museum documents the religious, ethnic and medical roots of the hospital and the surrounding neighborhood. Situated near the gift shop, it provides easy access for visitors who wish to view the historical items, including the highlight of the exhibit, the large (six feet in diameter) Holy Family stained-glass window, preserved from the chapel of the old hospital. Also among the exhibits are a fully costumed antique nun's habit on a mannequin, the hospital's first-day ledger, bricks from the second building, the original 1894 cornerstone, cornerstone materials from 1902, Sister Bernadette's baby bottle collection, old surgical tools, historic photos, medical instruments and other significant artifacts. The museum was featured in the November 1985 issue of *Catholic Health World*, a publication of the Catholic Hospital Association. Museum artifacts are also part of a historical collection on display at the American Hospital Association headquarters in downtown Chicago.

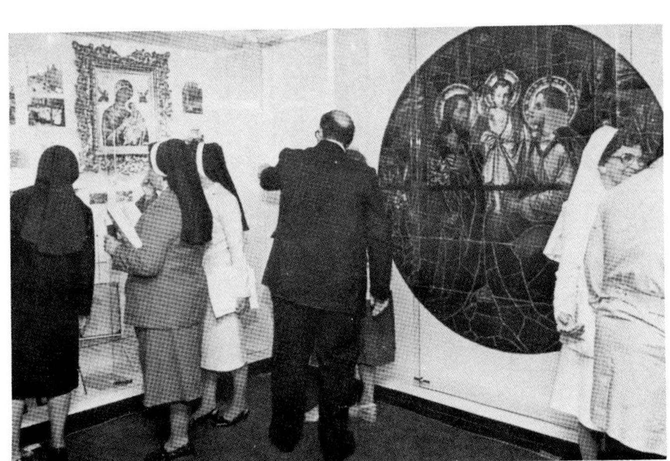

Sisters and friends of Saint Mary's toured the museum following opening ceremonies.

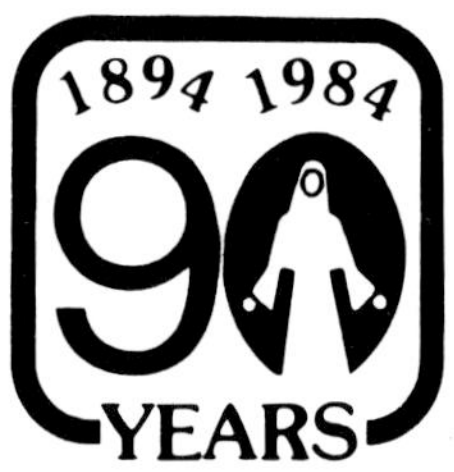

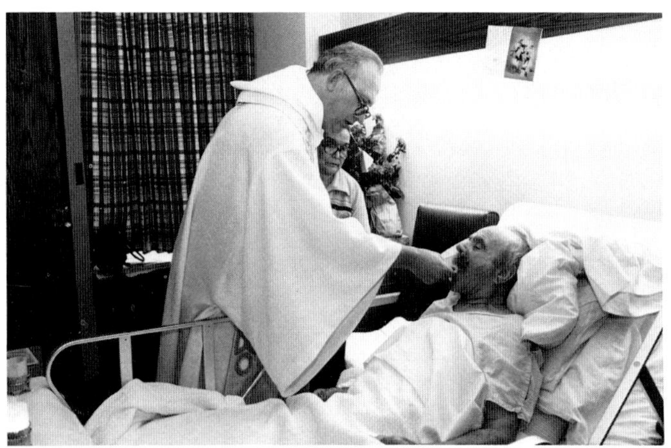

Father Lawrence Henry distributes communion to patients.

"Today, as always, the hospital is a haven for new Chicagoans on the city's near northwest side. With a devoted and distinguished medical/dental staff of 230, with 1,605 employees and with the latest medical facilities, Saint Mary's provides its patients with the newest, most advanced and sophisticated diagnostic, consultative and treatment services. ... Saint Mary's has grown with the city and the community it serves. It has undoubtedly contributed to the strength and cohesion of Polish culture in Chicago, an important segment in the rich mosaic of America's ethnic history. In its tradition of unselfish Christian service toward all races and creeds, Saint Mary's gives hope to all who enter its doors."

A continuing commitment to patient care

Bernard Henry, vice president of human resources, sits on the Guest Relations Committee chaired by Educational Coordinator Christine Waller, RN. Begun in 1988, the committee "finds ways to continually emphasize the importance of treating patients like guests," Henry says. "Our educational programs emphasize the principles we stand for: that everyone be treated with respect and dignity, that we'll

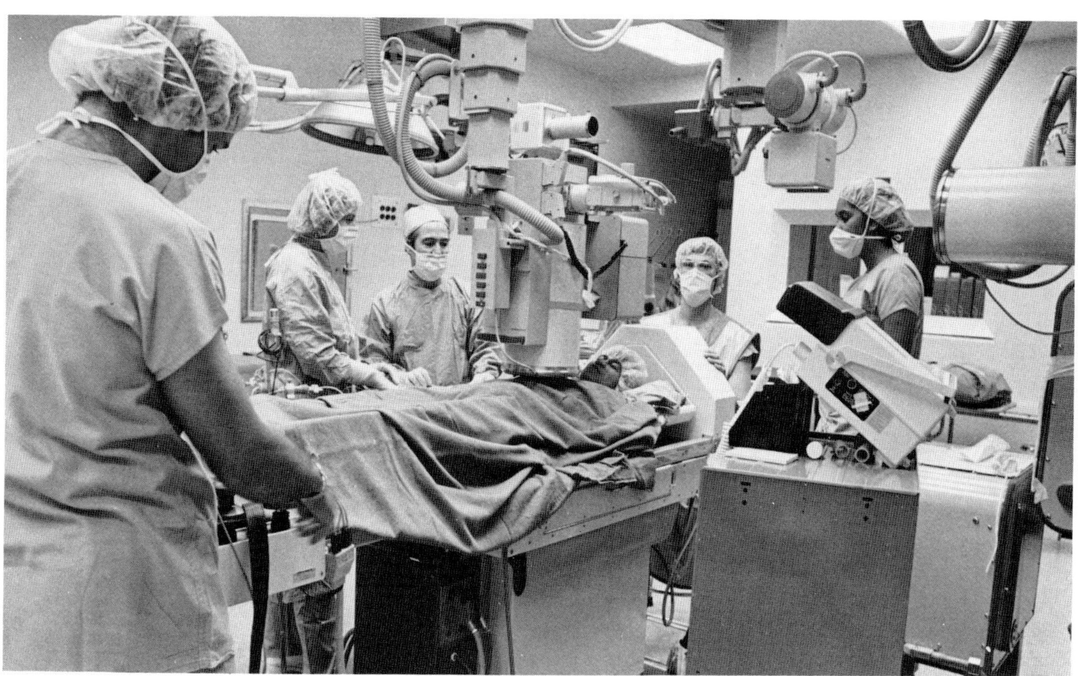

The Cardiac Catheterization program was expanded with new technology and space, 1989.

provide cost-effective services, that hospitality makes all the difference." Henry's duties as head of personnel, human resources development, volunteer services and security coincide with those aims. "We're always looking," he says, "to make a good fit in hiring. In the interview we ask how the prospect feels about our mission. We're an equal opportunity employer and we take great pains to make sure that everyone recognizes the nature of the institution and that we're really looking for people to contribute."

Janie L. Campbell, PhD, RN, is vice president, Patient Care Services. She believes that "nurses play a pivotal role in supplying essential patient care service in the hospital." Nursing is at the center of everything that happens to the hospitalized patient. While others—including the physician—come and go, nurses remain with the patient not only for specific professional nursing care, but to assure sequence, timing, continuity and implementation of the various services of the hospital and the medical cure plan of

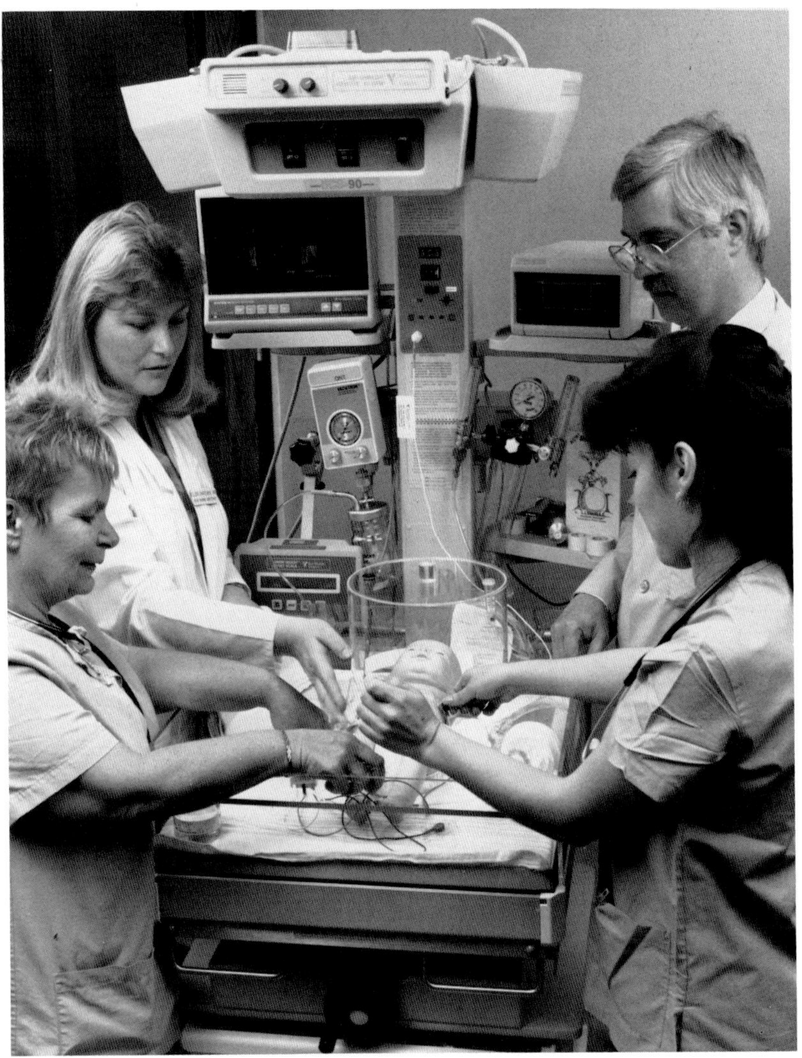

The 1990 Medical Staff Fall Benefit provided funds to expand facilities for high-risk pregnancies and newborns. With the new infant ICU system are (clockwise from lower left): Meredith Kramer, RN, maternity nurse; Ellen Zakrzewski, RN, maternity head nurse; Dr. Gerald Sunko, benefit chairman; and Cynthia Mayernik, RN, maternity nurse.

the physician. "The history of nursing at Saint Mary's," Dr. Campbell says, "is one of dedication to balancing requirements for technical expertise with the human dimension of caring for patients."

Nurses provide care to patients across a wide range of highly complex health conditions that require ever more extensive training and the acquisition of high-tech skills. They also coordinate all

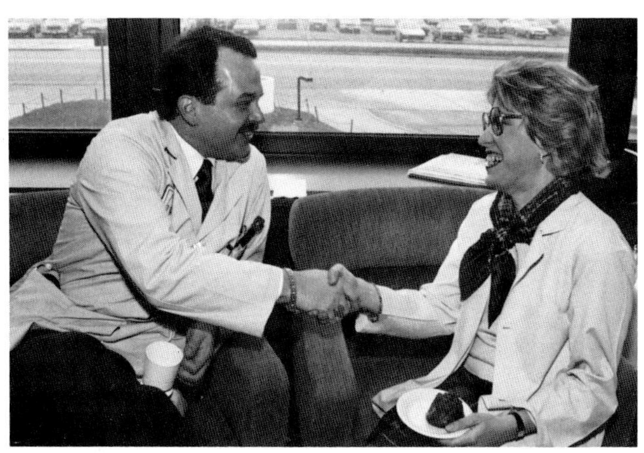

Dr. Bruce Becker and Dr. Janice Gilden

Bruce C. Becker II, MD, vice president, medical affairs and education, graduated from Saint Mary's Family Practice Residency Program in 1981 and remained at the hospital as assistant director of Medical Education. He has also held the positions of chairman of the Department of Family Practice and director of the Family Practice Residency Program. In addition to being a physician, he has earned several degrees, including a masters in health science administration. His wife, the former Irene Thibault, worked in Medical Affairs and Physician Relations at the hospital for 22 years.

"Saint Mary's Department of Family Practice, its Residency Program and the Family Practice Center, provide comprehensive medical care with particular emphasis on the family unit," said Dr. Becker. "The Center is the focal point for resident physicians during the three-year program. The family physician's continuing responsibility for healthcare is not limited by the patient's age or sex or by a particular organ system or disease entity. Through the Family Practice Center, each young physician builds a 'practice,' caring for more than 300 families in their final year of residency. A patient mix of medical, surgical, gynecologic, pediatric, obstetric, psychiatric and emergency cases provides the resident with a varied and full medical training experience."

Financial Management

Protection and careful appropriation of hospital resources requires sound financial planning if the hospital is going to meet its goals and objectives in support of its mission and strategic directions. The success of the strategic plan depends on its efficient deployment of its resources. Maintaining supervision over the hospital's financial areas in today's healthcare environment finds the issues of quality and financial health strongly related. 'Controlling costs should never be viewed as interfering with the delivery of good quality care,' says Senior Vice President and Chief Financial Officer Kenneth A. Kautzer. 'We accomplish both at Saint Mary's, even with a patient mix of 70 percent Medicare and Medicaid.' In 1993 over 70 percent of the hospital's total expenses of $102 million were controllable (i.e., salaries and wages, supplies, purchased services, etc.).

In support of the mission to render services to the sick, the needy and to the community in general, the hospital currently provides uncompensated care and service to the community in excess of $10 million each year. This amount is made up of charity care, community service, unreimbursed costs related to the Medicare and Medicaid programs, and other contractual arrangements.

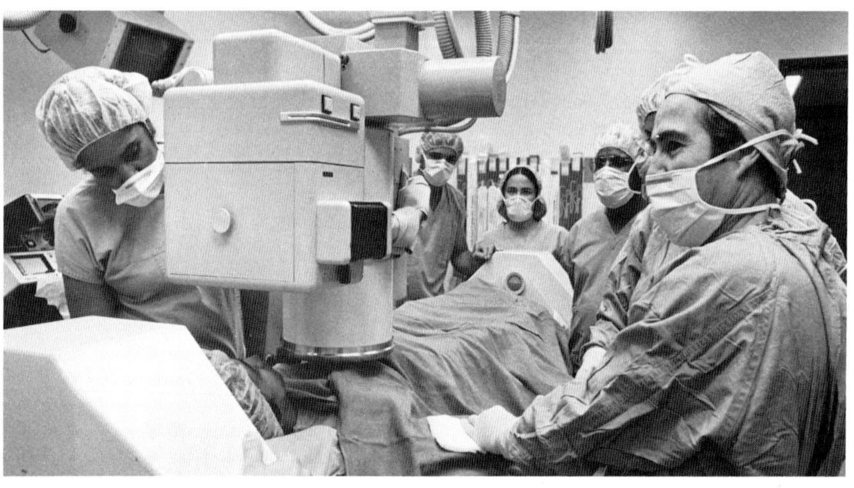

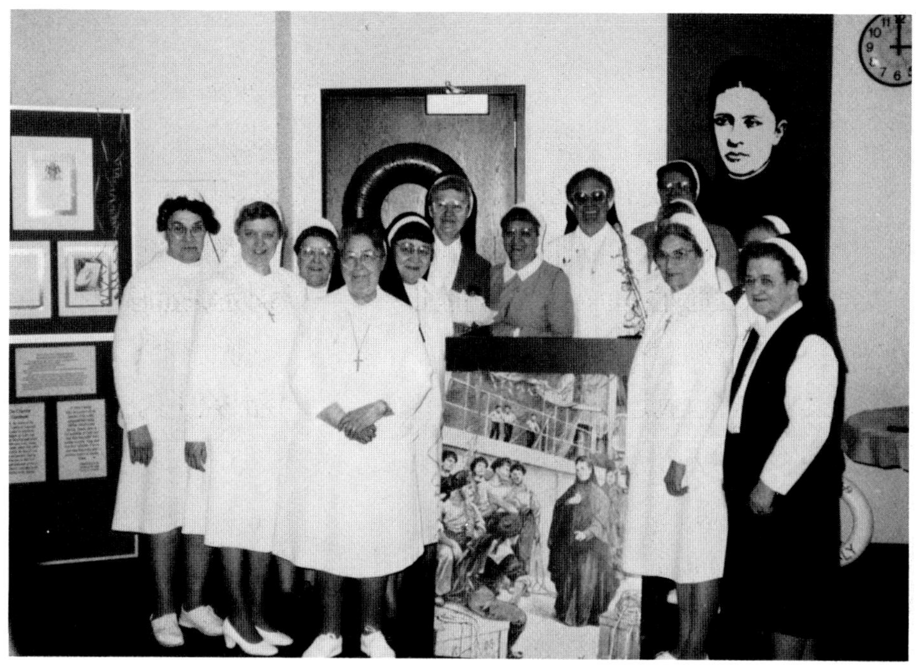

The Action '89 Committee sponsored a 'Bon Voyage' party for Saint Mary's Sisters. The Sisters were headed for Rome for the beatification ceremonies of Mother Foundress.

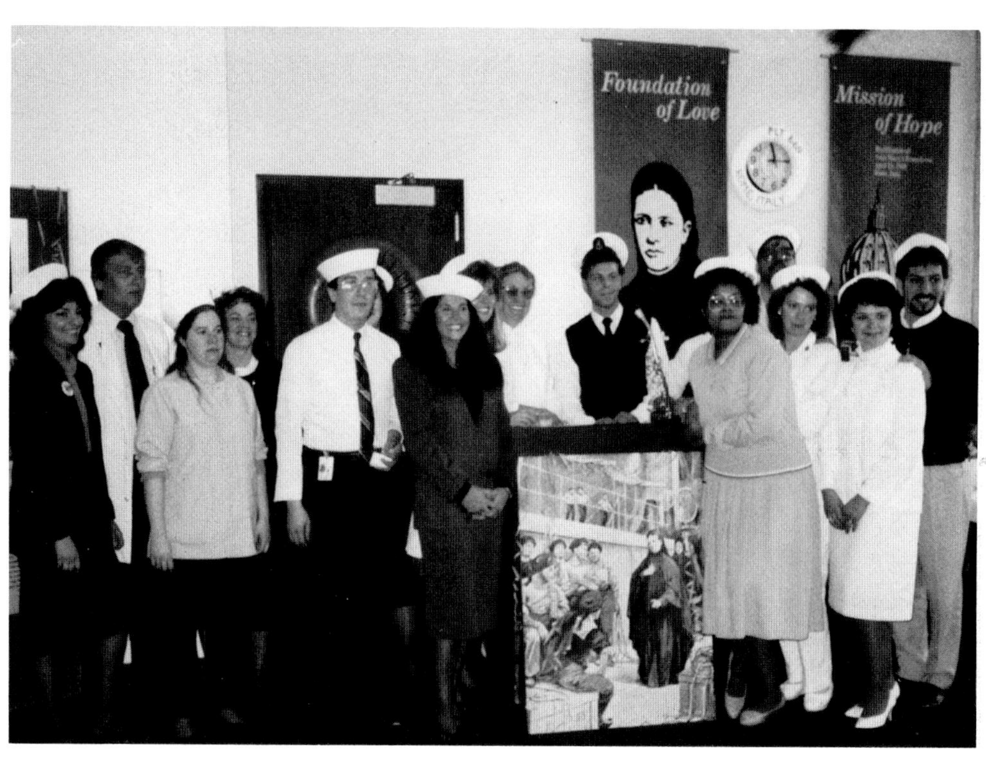

up and lets employees know what's happening throughout the building.

The Action Committee has sponsored a variety of events over the years. From arts and crafts shows and dinner dances to athletic and theater outings, the committee strives to promote varied activities to meet different

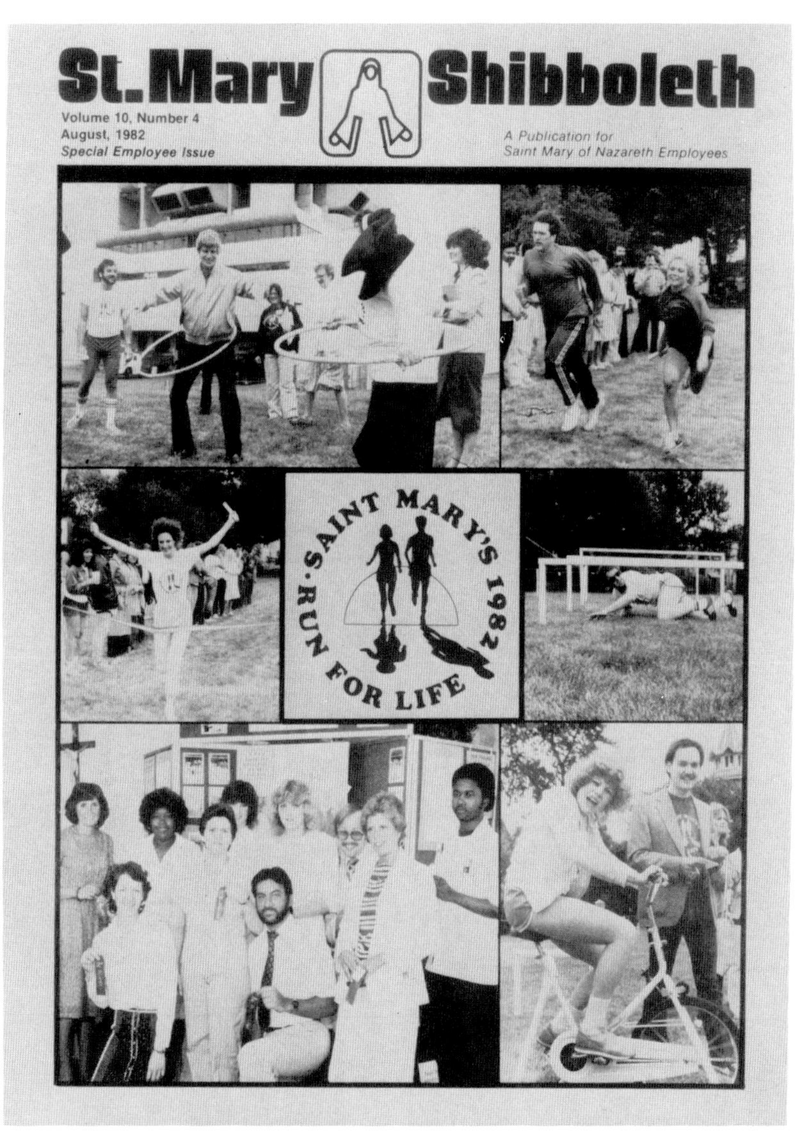

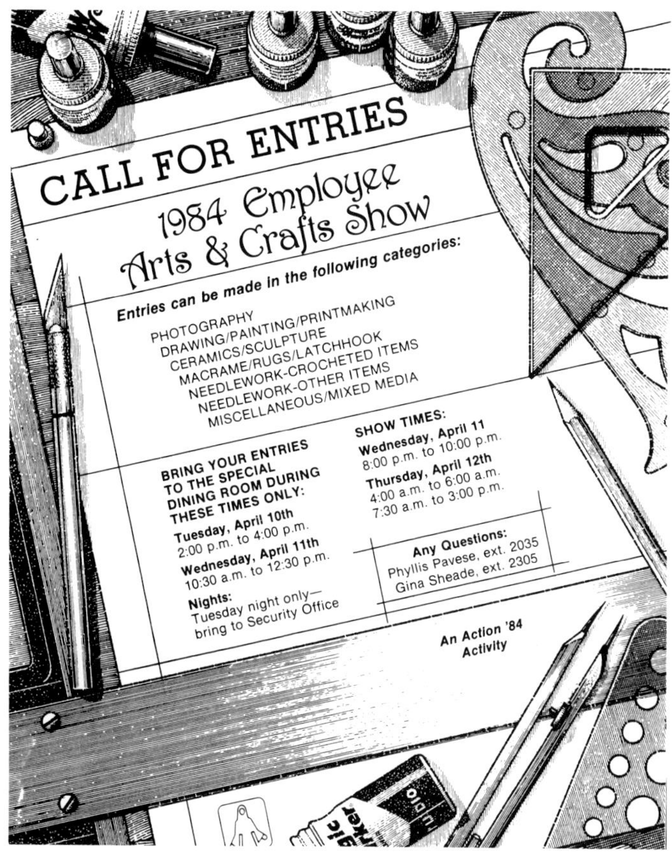

employees' interests. The Children's Christmas Party, held annually since 1982, is an afternoon of fun for the children of employees and medical staff. Several hundred attend each year. Run for Life, a "mini-Olympics" tied into the employee fund-raising effort, began in 1971 and continued until 1987.

Sister Kathleen describes the atmosphere in the old building as "much closer—it was smaller. When we moved to this new building, it was a culture shock. All of a sudden everything doubled. They hired a lot of people to take up the slack, and it took a long time to get to know everybody. The Action Committee helped keep Saint Mary's a family."

The employee payroll deduction fund drive annually nets $35-40,000 for various employee selected projects. Previous projects have included:

- The chapel stained glass window
- Employee cafeteria equipment
- CT Scanner
- Obstetrical equipment
- New mammography equipment

This employee commitment of support to their workplace is quite meaningful to foundations, corporations and other major donors.

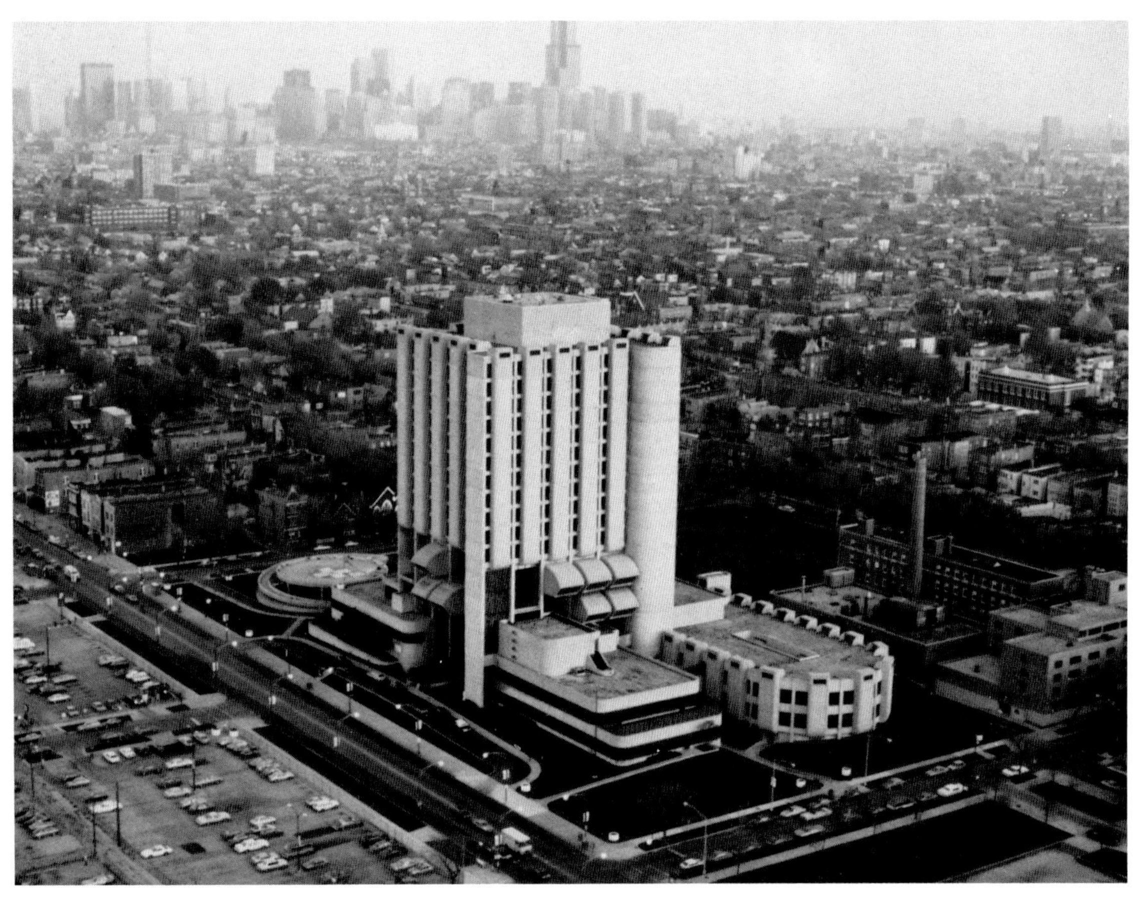

Caring for Children

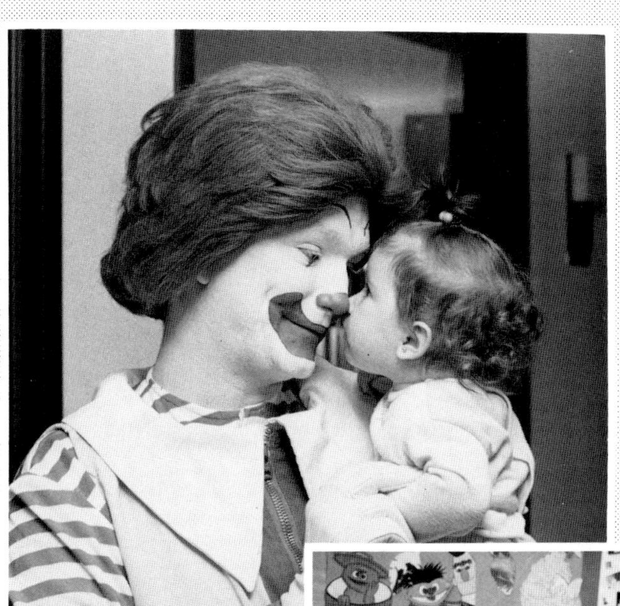

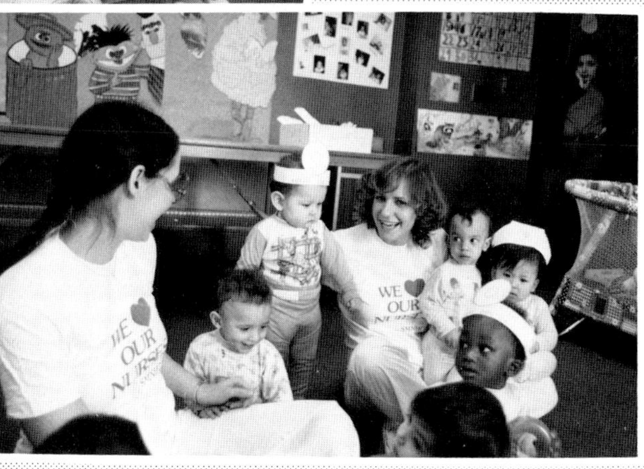

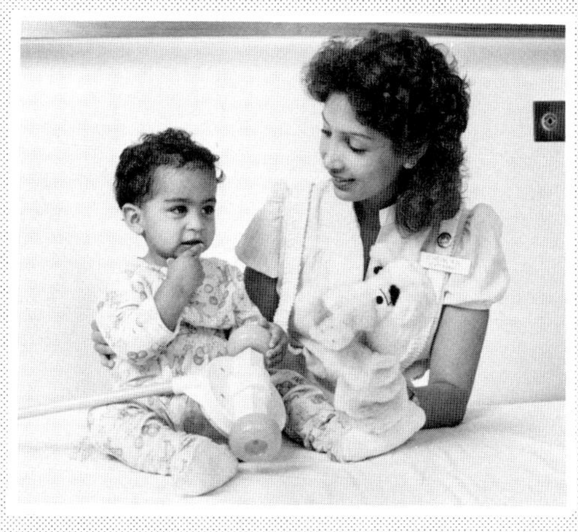

swing toward ambulatory care services and alternative delivery systems. To survive these pressures, we have had to change our service mix, our work volumes and our organizational structure twice over the last year."

The legacy of ever-increasing financial pressures from the 1980s has carried into the mid-1990s. At the end of this century, 50 percent of Americans will be middle-aged and elderly. Since these groups consume a large share of healthcare services, there will be significant changes in the demand for services. Elsa Goyma, RN, director of nursing for medical-surgical units, says she likes the universal access to healthcare in which each individual will receive a basic benefit package. "The concept of continuing coverage for the elderly will assist the individual to maintain his or her self-esteem and dignity," she says.

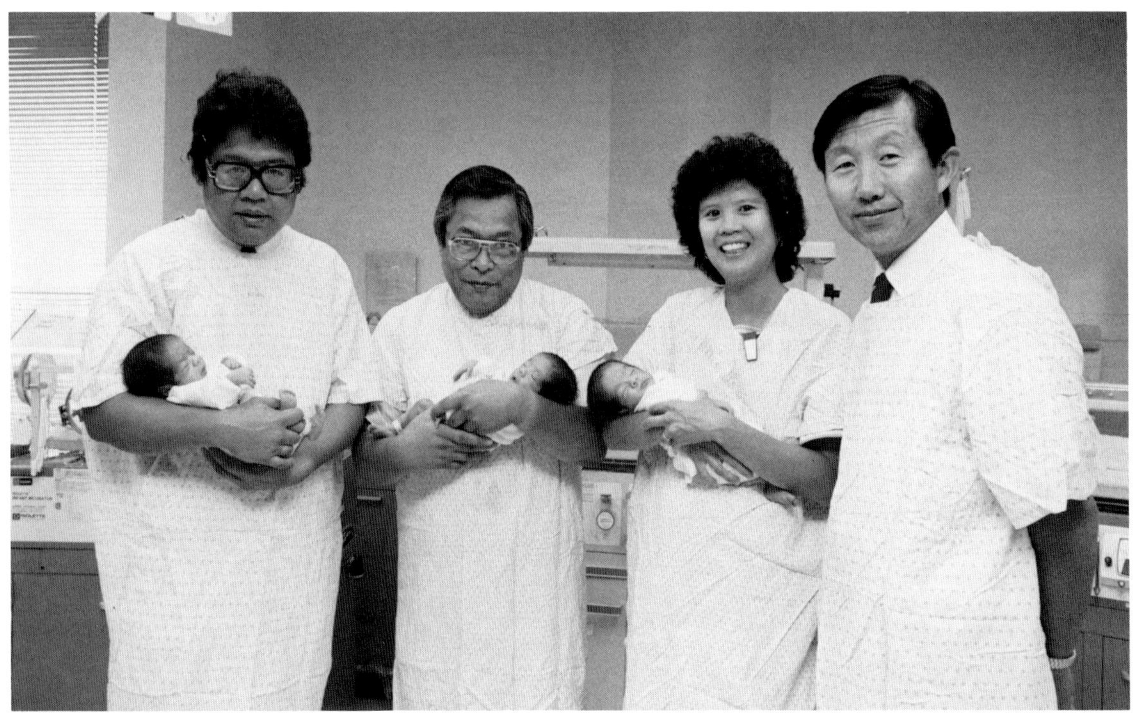

Caring for Children

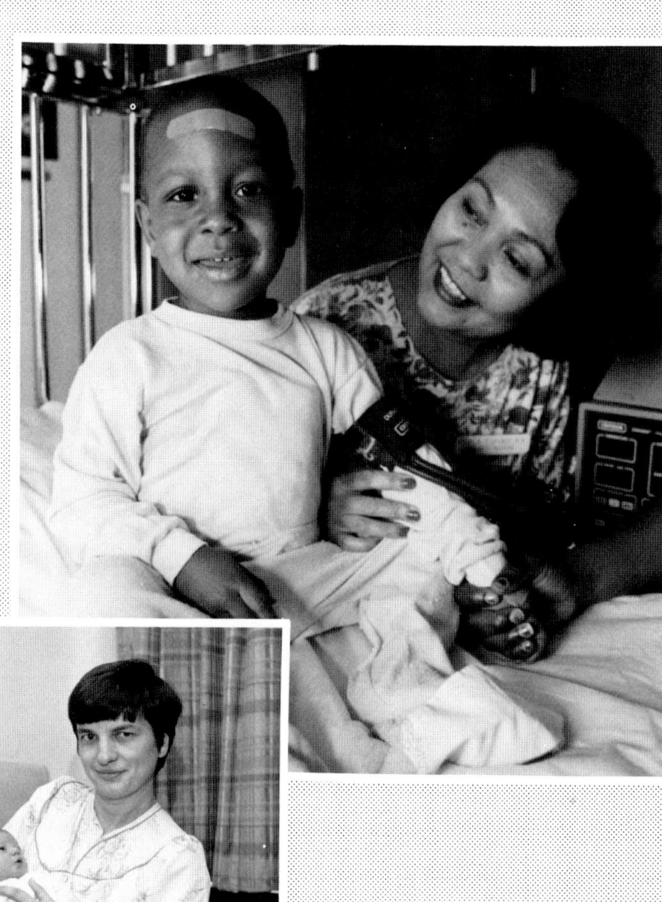

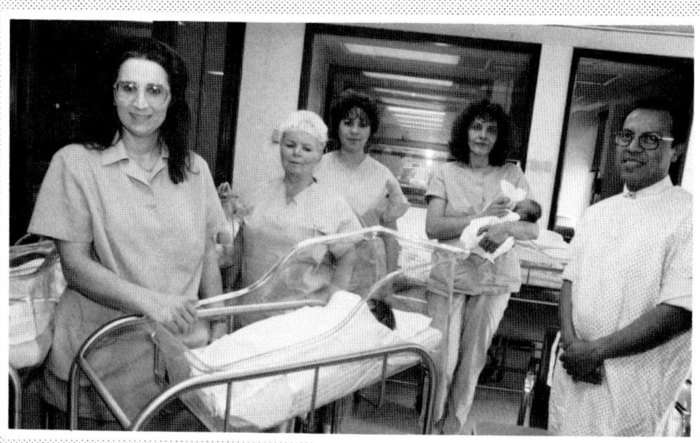

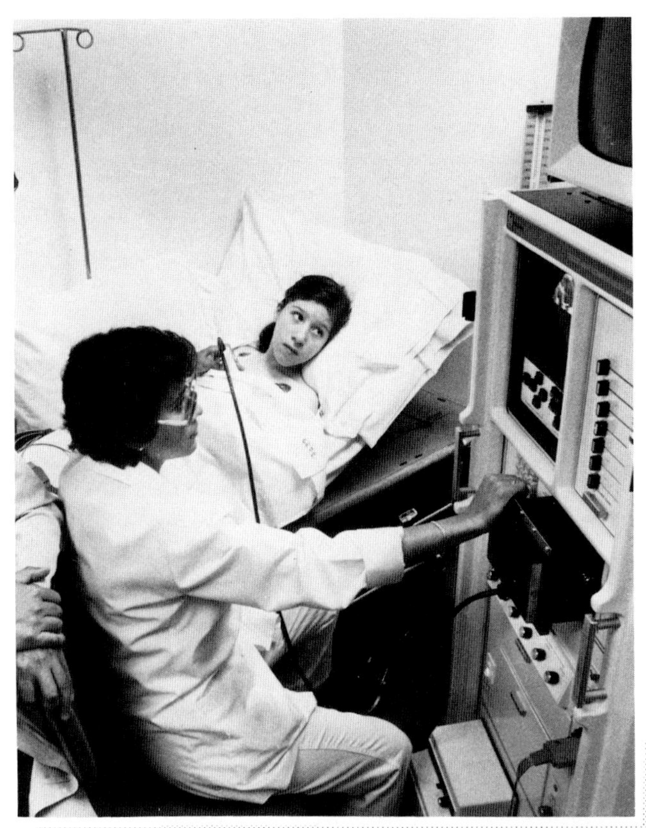

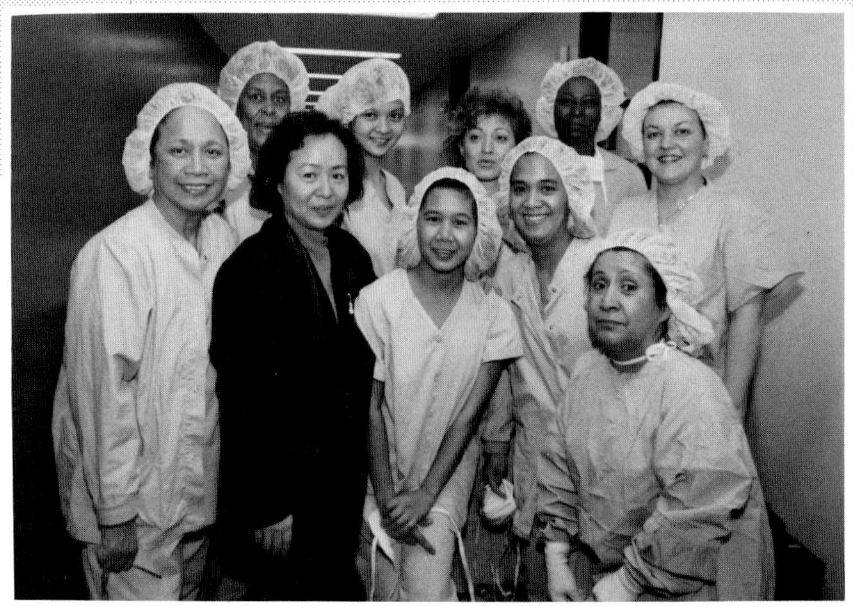

Saint Mary's People

Saint Mary's People

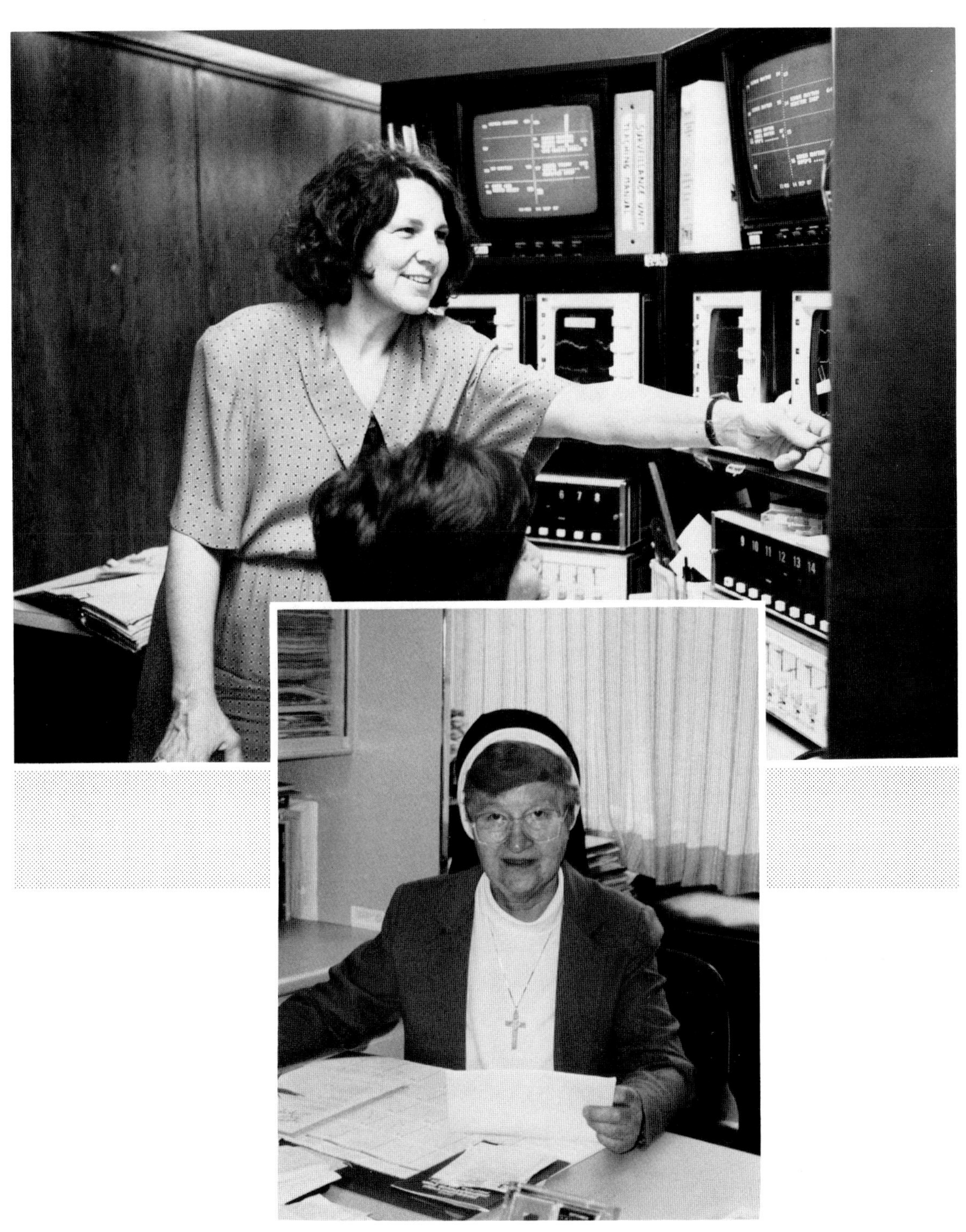

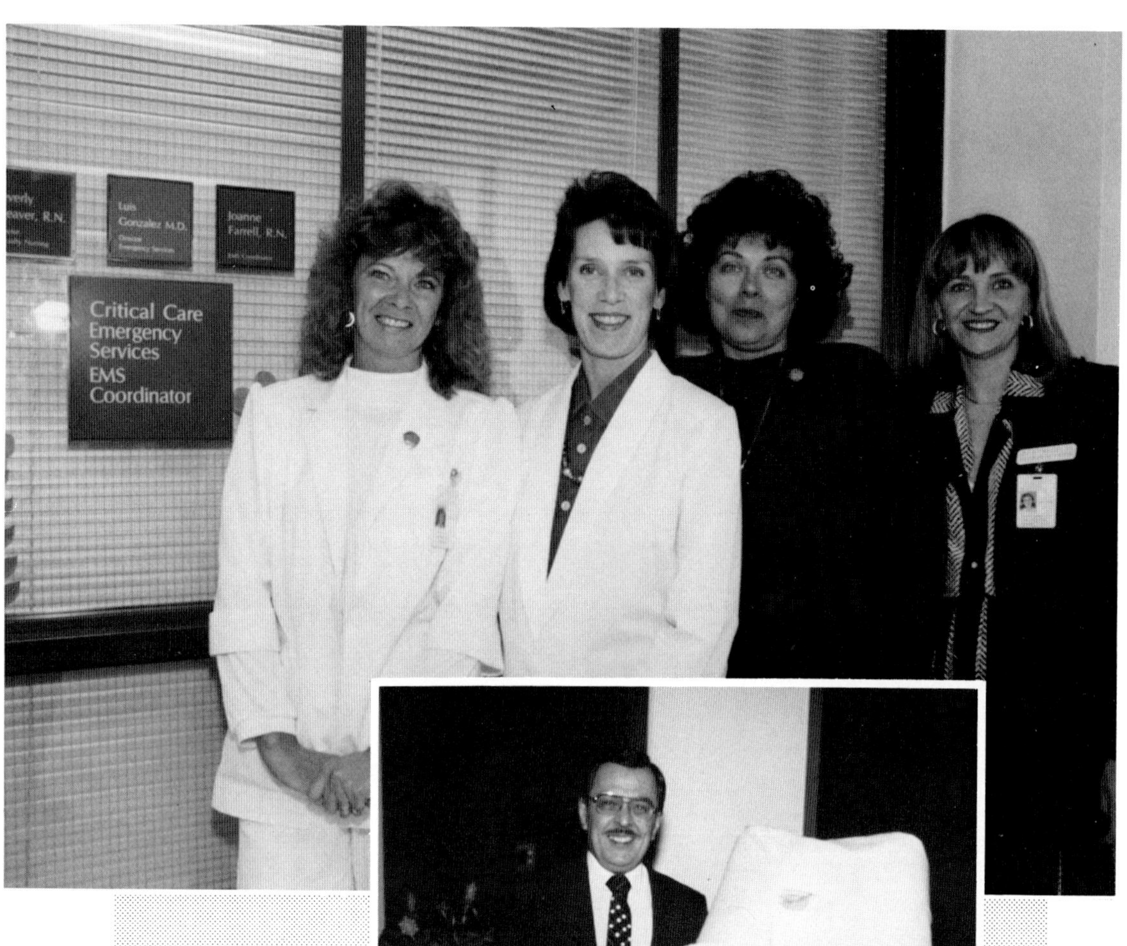

Saint Mary's People

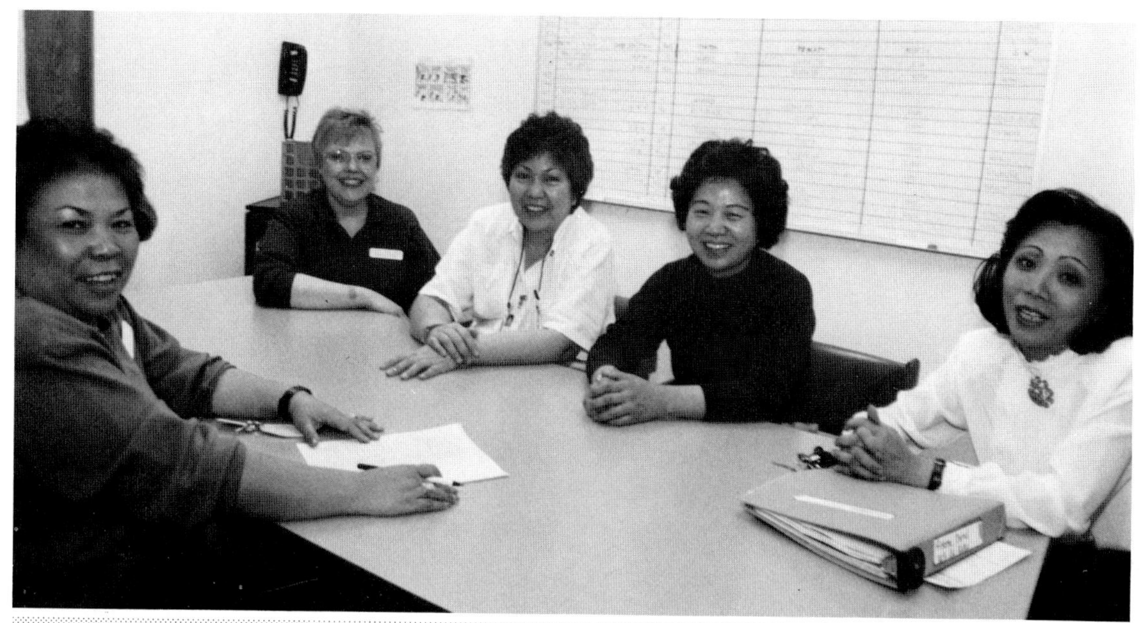

Saint Mary's People

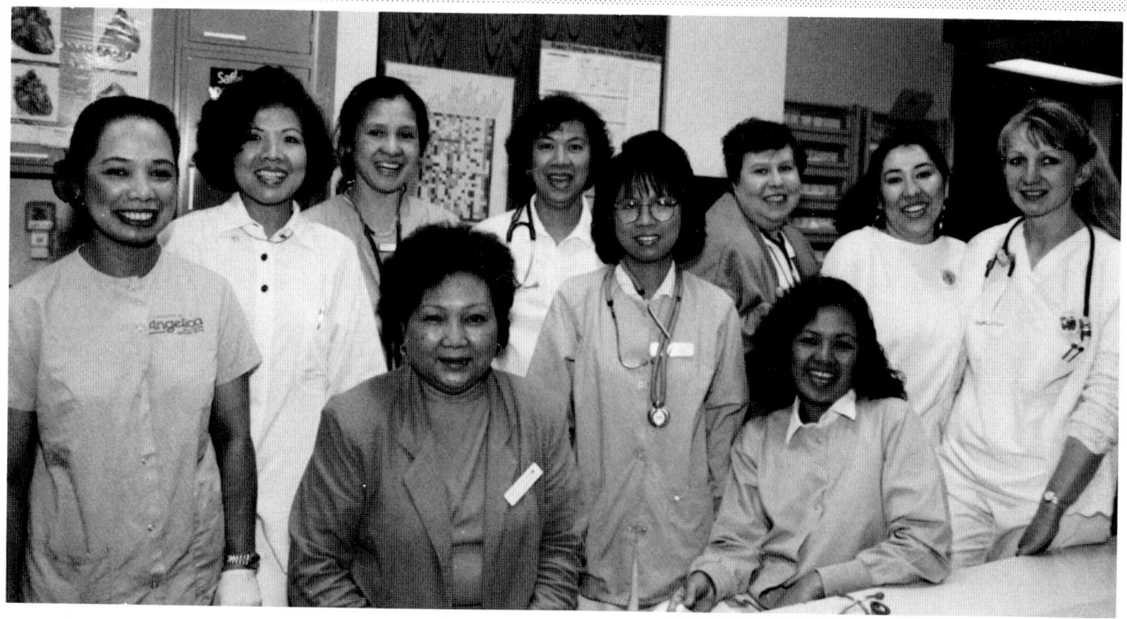

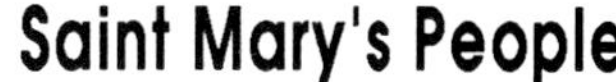

Saint Mary's People

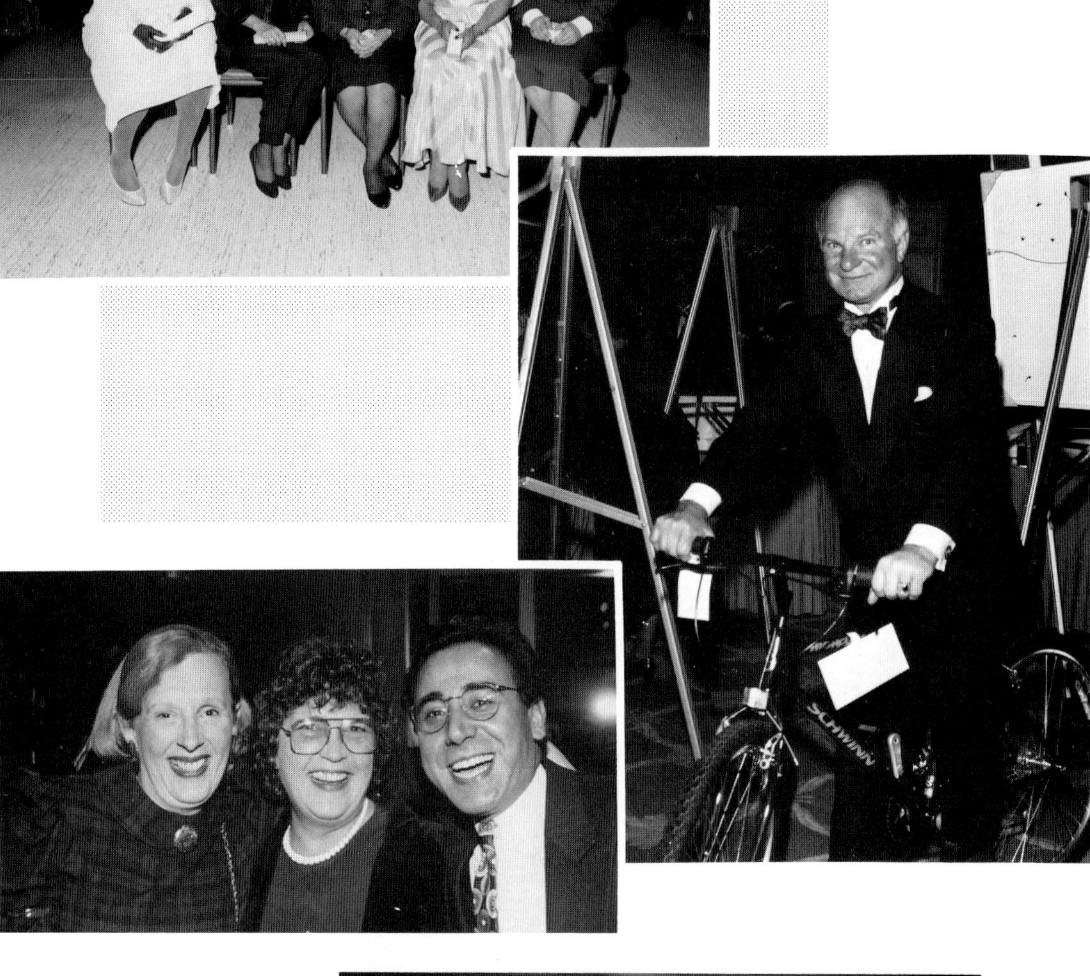

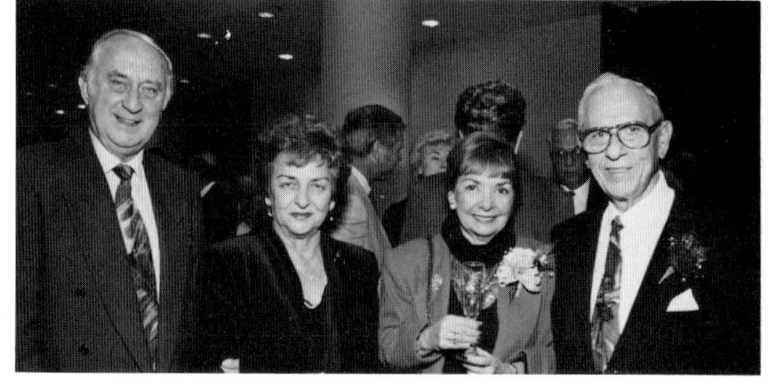

By the turn of the century, hospitals will devote fewer beds to patients who could recover more effectively at home. Those patients sick enough for hospitalization will be extremely ill and need resources devoted to specialized care. Acute-care facilities will be expanded to serve the needs of the older population. And as the population changes and healthcare reform occurs, so will the competitive environment. Saint Mary of Nazareth will be competing for patients with multi-hospital systems, HMOs and entirely new health organizations. The hospital may even become part of new alliances or networks.

Perhaps Dr. Sunko's predictions shed light on what will happen in other departments. "I would say in 10, 15 or 20 years radiation therapy would disappear as a science, that by then medicine will have direct ways with chemicals, antibodies or other agents attacking the tumors or finding them so early that radiation would be used less and less. I honestly think that radiation therapy might be de-emphasized by such developments in microbiology. ... As a resident I never thought there would be a cure for cancer. Now I've come to believe that in my lifetime we will see a cure for cancer or a major stride in its control. So instead of building a bigger department I would not be surprised if we became a smaller one."

"The complexity of hospital-medical staff interactions has resulted in new relationships over the past 100 years," says Dr. Bruce Becker. "However, the human relationship has remained unchanged. The demands for delivery of healthcare in the next century will realign the healthcare delivery team and result in relationships yet to be defined or imagined. Because the human relationship will remain unchanged, the future will remain bright. Our medical staff has always worked at strengthening this relationship between patient and healthcare provider. One hundred years ago, General Practice—or Family Practice—was the only type of medicine practiced, primarily due to limits of knowledge, lack of antibiotics and minimal technology. The generalists' forte was comforting an ill or dying patient. In 1994 medicine is embarking on a new frontier. The Human Genome Project, for example, will identify genetic tendencies to illness and disease that will allow medicine to drastically alter treatment protocols and methods. Yet the primary-care physicians' forte will still be to comfort and counsel the patient and family throughout the life process."

Tom Meirink says, "If you look at geographic dispersion of institutions in the Chicago area, there are 55 hospitals, about 100 in the metropolitan area. From a population density and economic perspective, Saint Mary's is situated just where it should be. I think our future is good—as a healthcare facility on the west side of Chicago—especially with healthcare reform on the horizon. We're replacing capital equipment that needs to be replaced. We're building. We're growing. We maintain and enhance skills. We take good care of our employees in terms of wages and benefits."

Saint Mary's has responded to the need for highly specialized, sophisticated tertiary-care services and offers a select number of such services. The hospital's competitive position is strong due to its reputation, carefully built over a century, for high-quality medical care provided in a Christian environment.

Wellness and family

"In the future," says Sister Stella Louise, "we need to move away from the model of the illness—even though we're a hospital—and focus more on health and wellness, the prevention of illness. We feel the future will concentrate on helping families come together again as we help them through their health-related difficulties. We have never emphasized family ministry as strongly as we are now."

Father Kobus agrees and speaks of the hospital family: "The Archdiocese needs to be always supportive of this ministry by priest personnel being present here. We have hope for the future that pastoral care will become more ecumenical. It comes about slowly. A lot of education needs to be done; a lot of walls need to be broken down."

The years ahead will witness new healthcare configurations and new ways to describe them: alliances, networks, groups, centers, sections, markets, and many more.

The hospital's sponsors, staff, and employees will meet the challenges of tomorrow as it has for a century: successfully.

The institution of Saint Mary's will evolve, while its mission will always be to offer the best medical care possible to all those in need of it, to emulate the healing ministry of Christ.

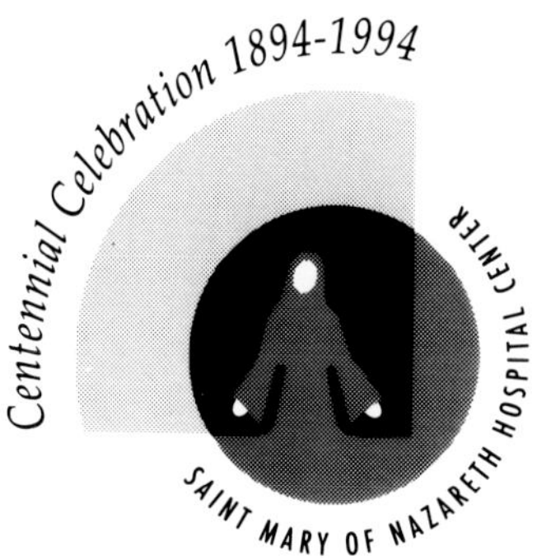

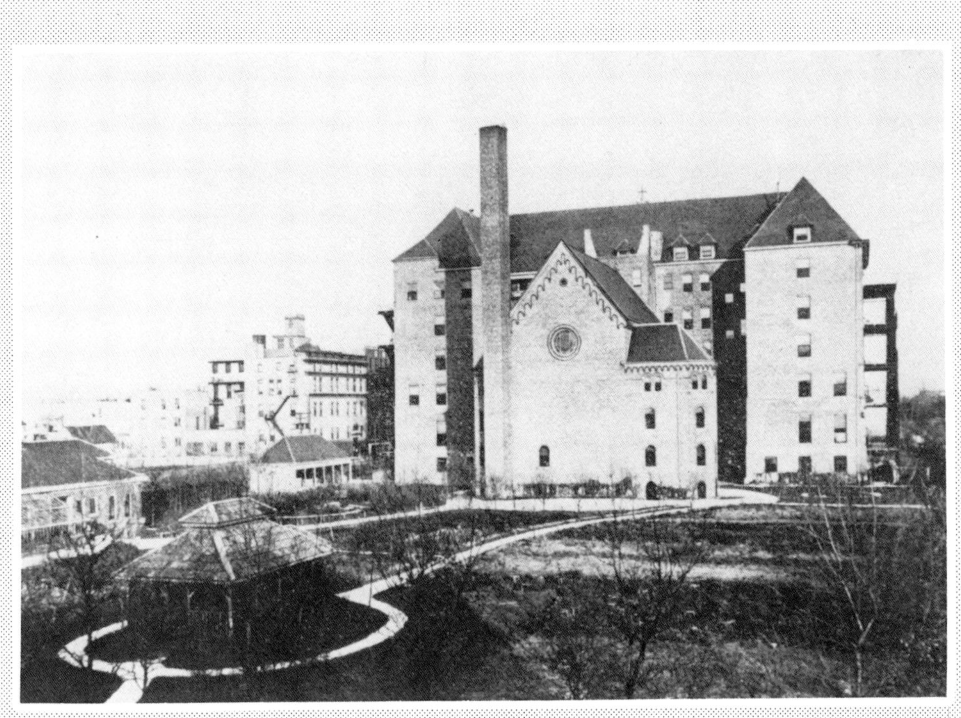

Saint Mary's in 1910, viewed from the west

The following is a selective list of milestones and other interesting trivia discovered during the research for this book.

1885 Mother Frances Siedliska and a company of 11 Sisters arrive in Chicago from Rome.

1889 Mother Frances entrusts the development of an appropriate hospital plan to Mother Mary Lauretta.

1894 April 10: The first official conference of the physicians favorably inclined towards the prospective hospital is held. In attendance: Doctors C.V. Midowicz, M. Janczewski, E. Czerniewski, R. Lande, W.A. Kuflewski, T. Kodis and Charles G. Davis. Dr. Davis is appointed president of the medical staff, and Dr. Kuflewski is appointed assistant surgeon.

The Governing Board is established and includes Mother Lauretta, Mother Paula and Mother Columba. Mother Paula becomes the hospital's first superintendent.

May 6: Holy Family of Nazareth Hospital opens.

Dire financial circumstances almost force the closing of the hospital, but financial contributions from the community and pledges of one year of free services provided by the medical staff help keep the doors open.

1900 A nurses' training school is established.
The first baby is born at the hospital.

1902 March 12: Doors open to the second Saint Mary's, 1120 North Leavitt Street.

A new instructional technique, the "clinical meeting," is introduced to Chicago by Saint Mary's and a few other hospitals. The meetings involve direct observation of clinical procedures by doctors and students.

1903 The School of Nursing graduates its first class consisting of seven students.

1904 November 16: The Women's Auxiliary of Saint Mary of Nazareth Hospital organizes.

1914 Electricity is installed.

1915 Saint Mary's becomes a founding member of the Catholic Health Association (CHA).

1917 The Sisters provide care to the employees of Corn Products Refining Company of Argo, Illinois, thus beginning their involvement in occupational health services.

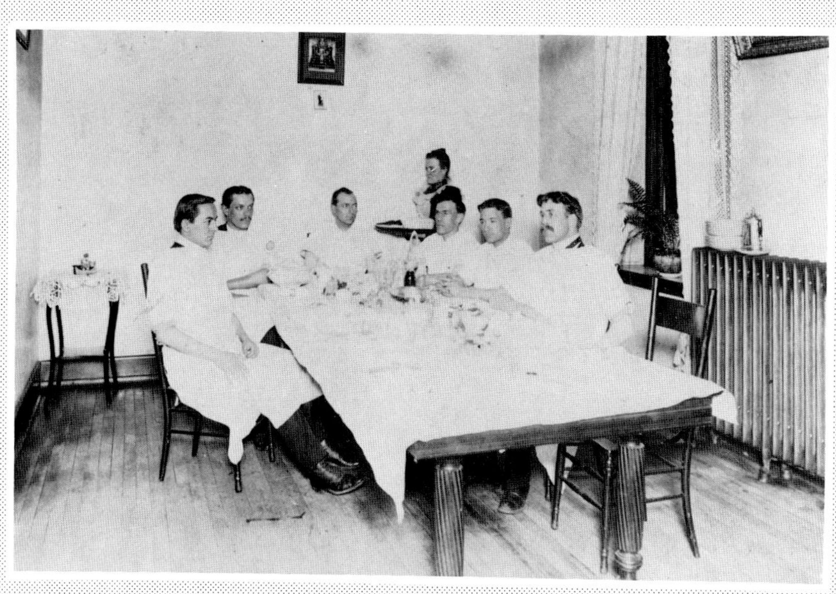

Physicians' dining room, about 1920

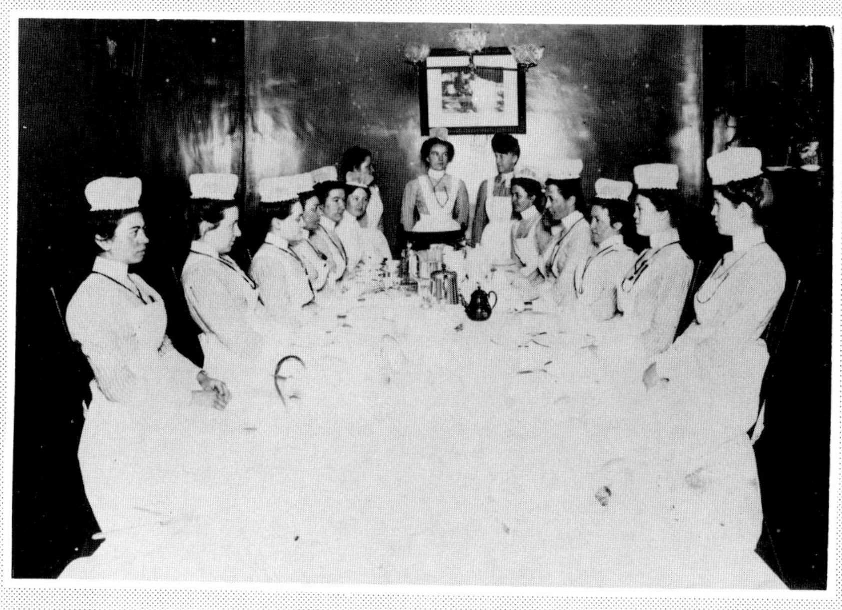

Nurses' dining room, about 1920

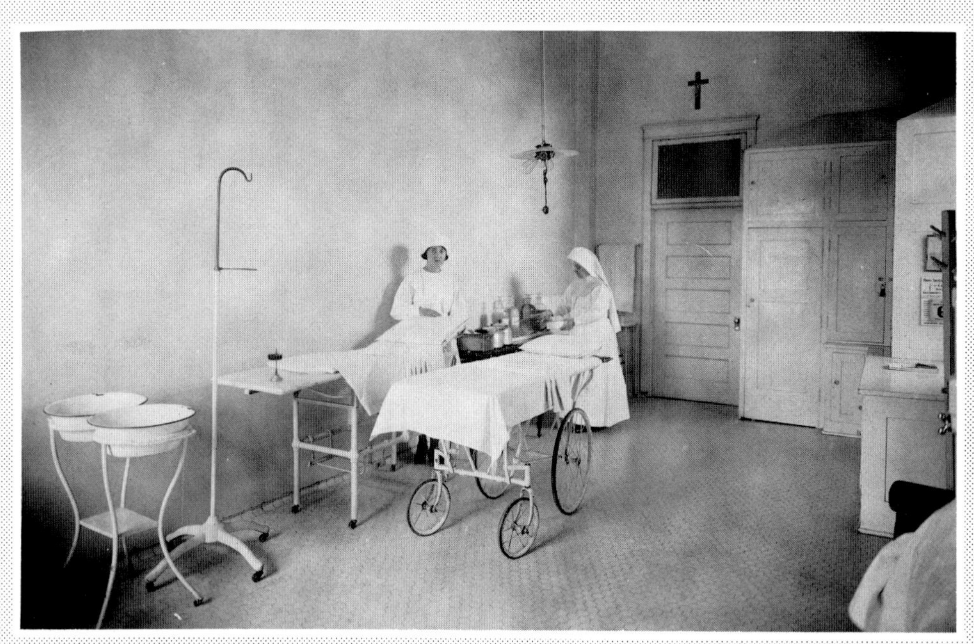

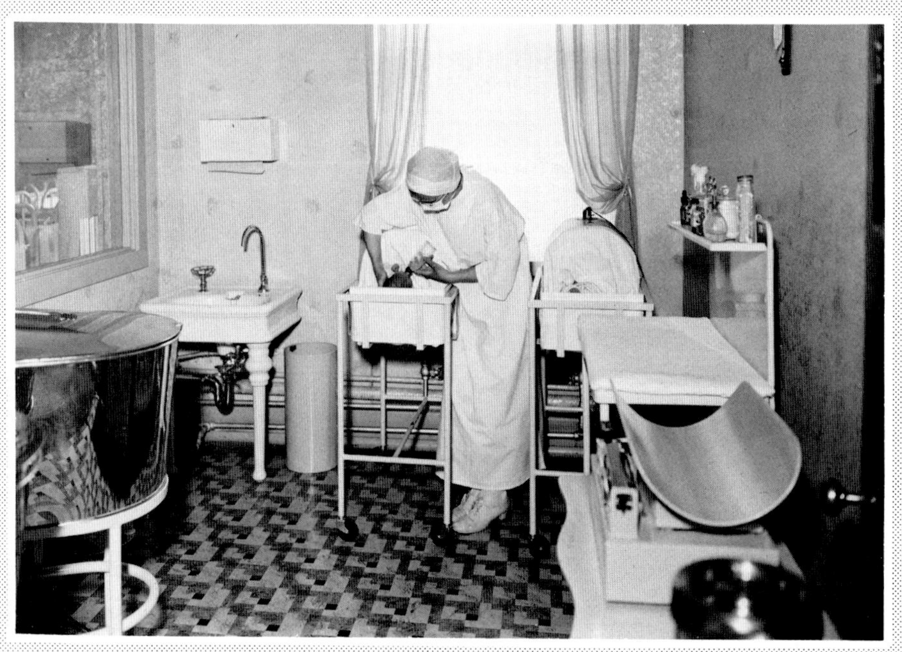

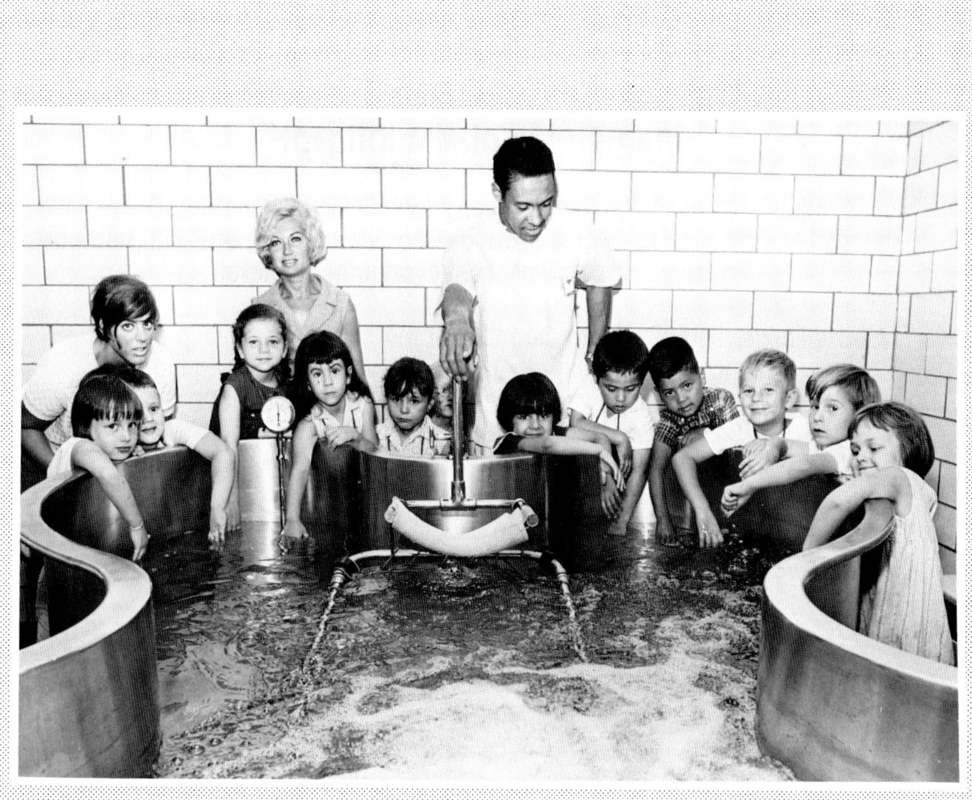

Physical Therapy Director Wendell Venerable demonstrates hydrotherapy equipment to Head Start students

1956 April 19: The 50,000th baby is born at Saint Mary's.

The School of Nursing is accredited by the National League for Nursing.

1959 Sister Mary Edelburg (Sister Stella Louise) becomes president of Saint Mary's.

1960 The Nursing Department institutes the Nursing Audit Committee (now known as the Quality Assurance Committee), under the direction of Sister Mary Agnes. This is one of the first quality assurance programs in existence.

Saint Mary's receives a letter from Poland addressed simply, "Polish Hospital, U.S.A."

1964 Sister Stella Louise, a founding member, is elected president of the Chicago Archdiocesan Conference of Catholic Hospitals.

A major three-year-long remodeling of the hospital is completed, increasing the capacity from 150 to 297 beds.

1965 The School of Radiologic Technology is affiliated with Crane Junior College in a three-year course of studies, the first such educational arrangement in the state.

1966

Approval by State of Illinois for the School of Nursing to condense its three-year program into a two-year sequence.

The emergency room cares for 9,600 patients.

Reorganization of hospital's top management and development of "functional management" takes place, whereby departments of similar function are grouped together under the direction of an administrator with expertise/background in that particular group function.

Wayne Hamilton establishes a centralized purchasing system with the actual buying of all hospital food, drugs, supplies and equipment accomplished by Purchasing Department buyers—a total materials management system.

The Cardiology Department performs several successful cardiac pacemaker implants. By the end of the year, it inaugurates electrocardiograms on the hearts of the unborn.

Banker Joseph Fitzer and attorney Mitchell Wiet are the first laymen added to the Governing Board.

Members of the Peace Corps visit Saint Mary's.

1967

The hospital establishes an intensive/coronary care unit and one of the city's first unit-dose medication dispensing systems.

1967-68

The purchase and subsequent razing of the former Lutheran Deaconess Hospital provides the site for the new Saint Mary of Nazareth Health Center Project.

1968

After a six-year lapse, training of interns is re-instituted with the approval of the American Medical Association.

Saint Mary's organizes the first mental-healthcare outpatient facility for community residents.

The hospital installs an electronic patient-data and hospital-information system, the first of its kind in Chicago and the third of its kind in the nation.

1969 Saint Mary's first Advisory Board is established, starting a tradition that would generate much-needed funds and goodwill for the hospital.

October: The medical staff holds its first Fall Benefit dinner dance at the Drake Hotel. Dr. John Meyenberg is chairman.

1970 The Woman's Board is established by Sister Stella Louise and Irene Allman.

Plans are announced to name the new facility's medical library for Hospital President Sister Stella Louise.

1971 January 1: Medicare introduces its new prospective reimbursement system based on diagnosis-related groups, "DRGs."

The Woman's Board sponsors its first benefit fashion show, raising $9,000 for Saint Mary's.

October: Entertainer Kaye Ballard is a special guest at the Medical Staff Fall Benefit.

1972 Mayor Richard J. Daley joins the Sisters in ground-breaking ceremonies for the new Saint Mary of Nazareth Hospital Center.

The Ruth and Frank Korte Family Care Center is established along with the Family Practice Residency Program.

1973 Saint Mary's is designated a comprehensive emergency facility under the Emergency Medical Service Plan.

SCAN (Suspected Child Abuse or Neglect) team is organized. Personnel includes members from Social Work, Pastoral Care, Mental Health, Maternity-Nursery, Nursing, Emergency, Pediatrics, Occupational Therapy and the medical staff.

1974

Saint Mary's Advisory Board holds its first Annual Recognition Dinner, honoring Illinois Secretary of State Michael J. Howlett.

Saint Mary's celebrates its 80th anniversary with a complement of nearly 200 dental and medical staff members and 1,050 employees.

1975

March 10: The new Saint Mary of Nazareth Hospital Center opens its doors.

The School of Nursing celebrates its diamond jubilee after graduating more than 2,300 nurses.

The hospital begins an oral surgery residency program in affiliation with Loyola University's School of Dentistry.

With a $500,000 grant from the Scholl Foundation, Saint Mary's establishes the Dr. William M. Scholl Orthopedic and Rheumatology Unit.

October: Talk-show host Phil Donahue attends the Medical Staff Fall Benefit.

Sister Janine and her dog help capture a theft suspect on Chicago's northwest side.

Saint Mary's becomes the first hospital in Chicago to adopt the Illinois Bell Telephone Company Centrex direct-dialing telephone system. The Women's Auxiliary assumes the complete cost of installing the Centrex system.

1976

The Cardiac Catheterization/Special Procedures Department opens.

Four physicians are the first graduates of the Family Practice Residency Program.

July 27: Demolition of the old hospital begins.

August 20: Saint Mary's is visited by Karol Cardinal Wojtyla, who will become Pope John Paul II.

1977

The hospital begins using computerized electrocardiograph system and provides access to the system by several other hospitals.

Ophthalmology service is instituted.

A computerized cardiac catheterization laboratory is established (the first hospital in Illinois), as is a full-service hyperalimentation nutritional support program (the first private hospital in the U.S.), under the direction of Mitchell V. Kaminski, Jr., MD

1978

An affiliation is forged with the University of Health Sciences/The Chicago Medical School, bringing medical students and resident physicians to train at Saint Mary's.

1979

A transtelephonic pacemaker monitoring service is made available to cardiology patients.

The first open-heart surgery is performed.

Saint Mary's enters into a full medical education program with the University of Health Sciences/Chicago Medical School. In coming years the hospital adds residencies in internal medicine, general surgery, psychiatry, family practice, and orthopedics.

Patient education is made available over the hospital's closed-circuit TV channels.

1980

Mitchell V. Kaminski Jr., MD, testifies on behalf of patients receiving intravenous hyperalimentation at home to the House Ways and Means Committee, Subcommittee on Health, in Washington, D.C.

August 2: A new record! Thirteen babies are born at the hospital between midnight and 6:20 p.m.

Saint Mary's and Harvard University co-sponsor a seminar on obesity in Chicago.

Anthony Silvetti, MD, presents a paper in England to the European Society of Parenteral-Enteral Nutrition, titled "Improved Wound Repair Through the Topical Application of Nutrients."

1980, Continued October: "I Dream of Jeannie" star Barbara Eden attends the Medical Staff Fall Benefit. She is the wife of then Advisory Board member and *Chicago Sun-Times* executive Charles D. Fegert.

1981

May 28: The School of Radiology graduates its last class of 23 students after 40 years of service. The school was the first in the Midwest to combine hospital/college cooperation in an associate degree program.

In June the first corneal transplant at Saint Mary's is done by Philip Konecny, MD.

A Cardiac Rehabilitation Program, conducted by Salvatore A. Motto, MD, is approved for patients with heart problems. It focuses on closely monitored exercise and nutrition for the cardiac patient.

1982

The hospital acquires a computerized tomography (CT) whole body scanner, substantially expanding the staff's ability to diagnose certain illnesses and injuries.

Dr. Anita Johnson is elected first female president of the medical staff.

1983

The Lifeline Program is instituted under the direction of Volunteer Services director Mary Uhrick. This personal emergency response system connects elderly and disabled people to Saint Mary's via a wireless transmitter and telephone.

May 4: Joseph Cardinal Bernardin becomes the 10th Advisory Board Recognition Award recipient.

Saint Mary's receives a three-year, National Cancer Institute grant, which facilitates treatment of certain cancer patients with new and experimental drugs. The hospital is one of only 59 hospitals and doctor groups to receive such a grant, which allows people to be treated in their own communities rather than at distant university medical centers.

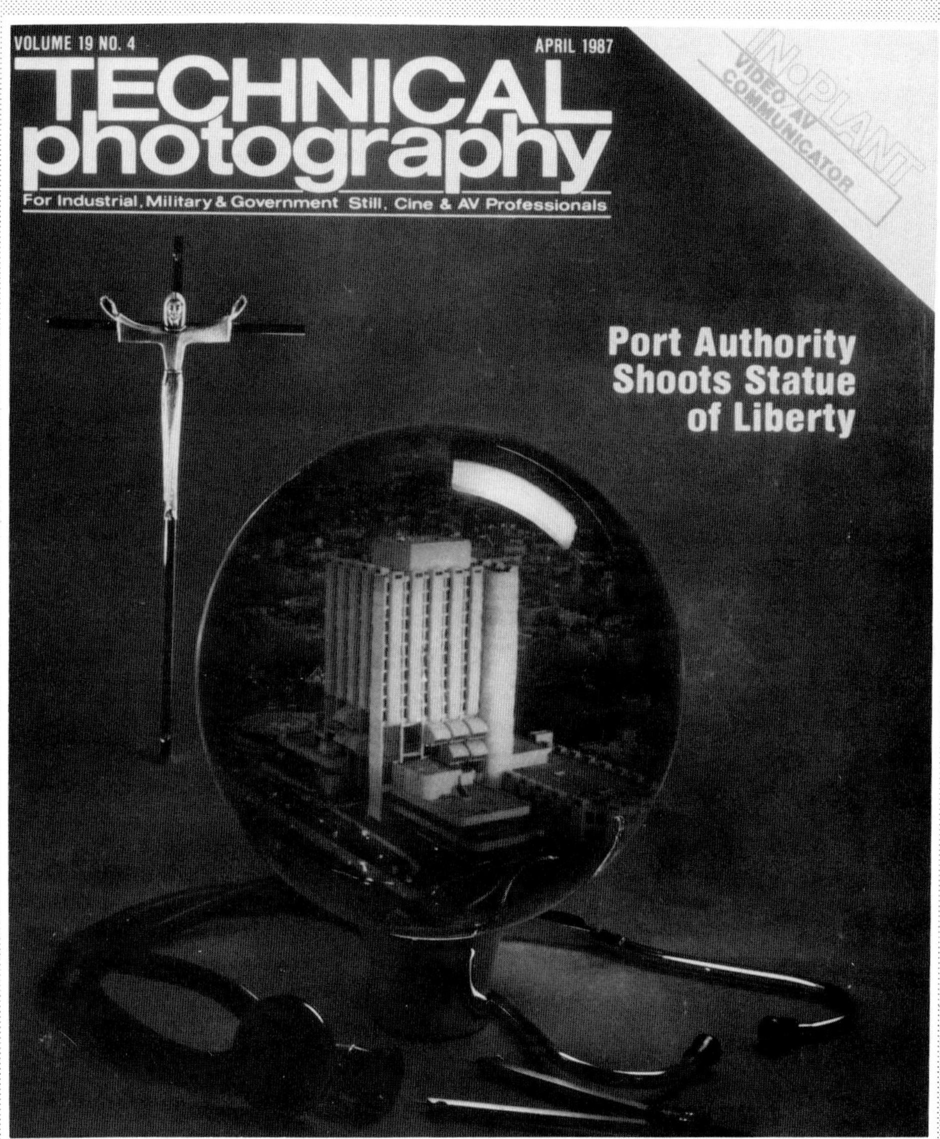

Saint Mary's 1985 annual report was featured on the cover of the April 1987 issue of *Technical Photography* magazine.

The cover, 'Charting a course for the future,' was created by staff photographer Curt Cechowicz, Media Services, and Phyllis Pavese, Public Relations.

1984

MedStar, Saint Mary's aero-medical emergency helicopter service, provides emergency transport to a three-state area within 150 miles.

Closed-circuit TV provides patient information programs in Spanish and Polish, in addition to English.

Saint Mary's purchases a satellite building on Belmont, near Central Avenue, from which Saint Mary's Home Health Service, hospital pre-admission testing and clinical laboratory outreach services will operate.

The Sisters of the Holy Family of Nazareth celebrate 100 years in America. In celebration, Saint Mary's opens its historical museum and the Congregation receives the 1985 Recognition Award.

1985

Home Health Services and the JOBMED occupational medicine program begin operation.

The Illinois Chapter of the American Society of Heating, Refrigerating and Air Conditioning Engineers (ASHRAE), awards the hospital its first place energy conservation award.

September 24: Chicago Auxiliary Bishops Plácido Rodríguez and Alfred Abramowicz participate in the dedication of the newly constructed helipad.

1986

The School of Nursing closes.

"Medical Minutes"—aired for 52 weeks on "Good Morning, America," "The Today Show" and "Eyewitness News." TV info-mercials promoting Saint Mary's as a critical-care center to more than 1,000,000 viewers.

The Maternity Savings Plan is launched.

May: Chicago Bears' Head Coach Mike Ditka receives the 1986 Advisory Board Annual Recognition Award.

1987

January 8: Father Walter Krempka dies after over 26 years as hospital chaplain and friend of Saint Mary's. Previously, he served as Associate Pastor of St. Mary of Perpetual Help, St. Fidelis, and Immaculate Conception Parishes. In 1960 he joined Saint Mary's pastoral care staff.

A diabetes education center is established to help diabetics better cope with their chronic illness.

The Adolescent Psychiatric Treatment Unit is opened on the 15th floor, a unit for adolescent patients suffering from behavioral disorders as a primary diagnosis.

Saint Mary's opens "MedStop" medical clinic on the southwest side.

Michael R. Quinlan, president and CEO of McDonald's Corporation, is the Recognition Award recipient. Ronald McDonald pays a surprise visit to Saint Mary's patients and employees.

The Illinois State Police Director's Award of Merit is presented to the doctors, nurses and staff, "In recognition of dedication and professionalism displayed during the emergency treatment of Illinois State Trooper Dennis M. Galle #3614, who was a victim of a gunshot wound on July 18, 1987. Your outstanding and unselfish efforts resulted in saving the life of the officer."

1988

Spanish and Polish language day hospital services are established for mental health center patients.

1989

February 11: Saint Mary's loses its director of pharmaceutical services and local superior, as Sister Lucille is elected Provincial Superior of the Sacred Heart Province.

April 23: In a ceremony at Saint Peter's Basilica in Rome, Pope John Paul II beatifies Mary of Jesus the Good Shepherd, Frances Siedliska, Foundress of the Congregation of Sisters of the Holy Family of Nazareth. The Sisters reaffirm their dedication as a Congregation to the moral and religious renewal of family life as the central focus of their ministry.

The Governing Board

Chairpersons

Mother Lauretta Lubowicka
1889-1895, 1896-1903

Mother Columba Trzewiczek
1895-1896

Mother Sophia Kulawik
1903-1918

Mother Antonia Danisch
1918-1925

Mother Ignatius Romanowska
1925-1931

Mother Regina Wentowska
1931-1938

Mother Richard Rutkowska
1938-1947

Mother Aloysius Kozlowski
1947-1959

Mother Getulia Honorowski
1959-1965

Mother Gloria Madura
1965-1971

Mother Alexandra Budzinska
1971-1979

Sister Hilary Dyrcz
1979-1983

Sister Loretta Markiewicz
1983-1989

Sister Lucille Madura
1989-

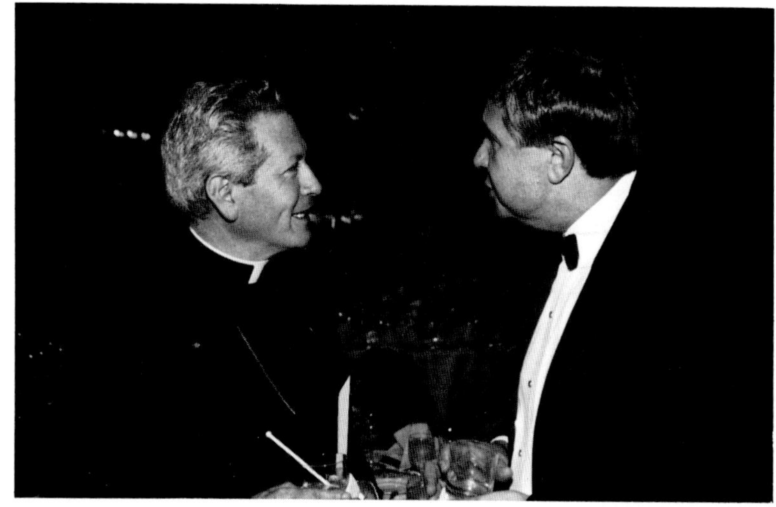

Governing Board member Bishop Plácido Rodríguez, CMF, (left) and Director of Pathology Laboratories John T. Preston, PhD, attend a hospital benefit.

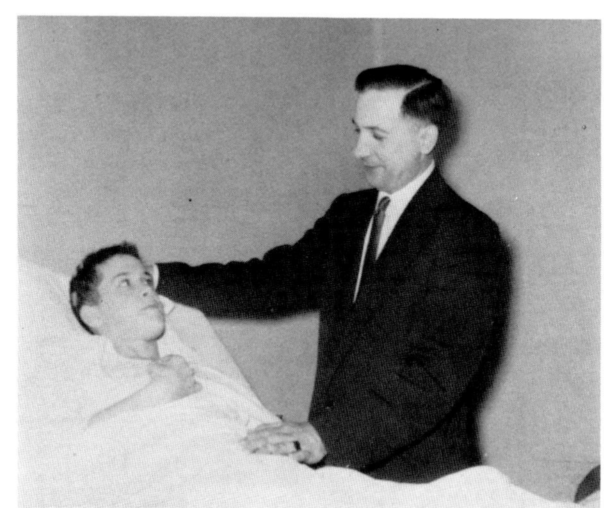

Dr. Preston's father, John B. Preston, MD, was a general surgeon at Saint Mary's from 1950-1958.

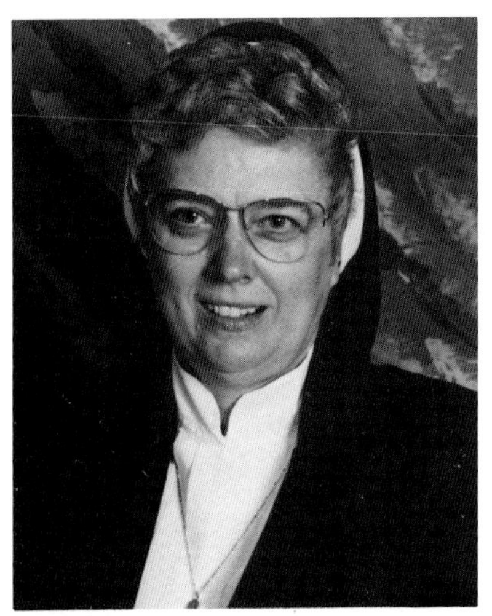

Sister Lucille Madura, Chairperson, Governing Board

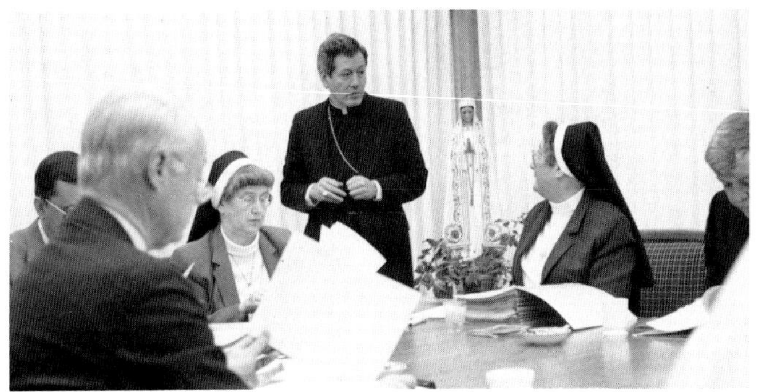

Governing Board meeting, 1988

1994 Governing Board

Sister M. Lucille, CSFN
Chairperson

Eugene P. Mroz
Vice Chairman

Sister M. Amata, CSFN
Sister Kathleen Ann, CSFN
Sister Marie, CSFN
Sister Rose Marie, CSFN
Sister Sally Marie, CSFN
Sister Stella Louise, CSFN
Sister M. Virginia, CSFN
Sister Virginette, CSFN
Stanley Gradowski
Nam S. Huh, MD
Walter M. Kelly Jr.
William V. Mollihan, MD
James Phillips
Lawrence Ptasinski
Most Rev. Plácido Rodríguez, CMF

Life Trustees

Edward J. Allman
Allwyn Baptist
King Deets, PhD
E.M. 'Mick' Donahue
Joseph Fitzer
Anita Johnson, MD
Jack C. Leahy
Michael E. Luby
Stephen A. Malato, Sr.
John C. Meyenberg, MD
Salvatore A. Motto, MD
Donald C. Romans
Anthony R. Sapienza, MD
Constantine Tatooles, MD
Mitchell J. Wiet

Sisters at Saint Mary of Nazareth

Sister Kathleen Ann, CSFN,
Superior
Sister M. Agnes, CSFN
Sister Ann Marie, CSFN
Sister M. Anne, CSFN
Sister M. Antonia, CSFN
Sister M. Aquinas, CSFN
Sister M. Barbara, CSFN
Sister M. Bernadette, CSFN
Sister M. Blanche, CSFN
Sister M. Clotilde, CSFN
Sister M. Constance, CSFN
Sister M. Dorothy, CSFN
Sister M. Eugene, CSFN
Sister M. Floriann, CSFN
Sister M. Gabrielle, CSFN
Sister Helen Marie, CSFN
Sister Rita, CSFN
Sister Rose Marie, CSFN
Sister Stella Louise, CSFN
Sister M. Sylvia, CSFN
Sister M. Valentine, CSFN
Sister M. Violet, CSFN

Medical Staff Leadership

Chiefs of the Medical Staff

1894-1896	Charles G. Davis, MD
1896-1925	Albert J. Ochsner, MD
1925-1937	Stephen R. Pietrowicz, MD
1937-1943	George R. Mueller, MD
1943-1950	Thaddeus Larkowski, MD
1950-1960	Edward Warszewski, MD

Presidents

1934	Stephen R. Pietrowicz, MD
1935	Leo M. Czaja, MD
1936	D. Phillips, MD
1937-38	Peter J. Orzynski, MD
1939	William McCabe, MD
1940	Leon Grotowski, MD
1941	Peter J. Doretti, MD
1942	Bernard C. Kolter, MD
1943	E. Johannes, MD
1944	W.A. Kuflewski, MD
1945	Thaddeus Larkowski, MD
1946	Casimir F. Przypyszny, MD
1947	P. Czwalinski, MD
1948	Joseph Welfeld, MD
1949	Florian Ostrowski, MD
1950	Peter J. Orzynski, MD
1951	John F. Tenczar, MD
1952	Maurice F. Snitman, MD
1953	Frank Mackowiak, MD
1954	Joseph G. Hillebrand, MD
1955	Frank J. Piszkiewicz, MD
1956	Chester J. Challenger, MD
1957	Joseph S. Drabanski, MD
1958	Nicholas A. Casciato, MD
1959	Mitchell Krupinski, MD
1960	Salvatore A. Motto, MD
1961	Edward J. Swastek, MD
1962	Michael Kutza, MD
1963	Joseph Kostrubala, MD
1964	John F. Wiet, MD
1965	Salvatore A. Motto, MD
1966	Joseph Strzyz, MD
1967	Michael Giannini, MD
1968	John C. Przypszny, MD
1969-70	John E. Meyenberg, MD
1971-72	Conrad Wiet, MD
1973-74	C. Dereng, MD
1975-76	Bruce P. Zummo, MD
1977	John E. Meyenberg, MD
1978	Walter Cebulski, MD
1979	Donald C. Wharton, MD
1980	Walter Kawula, MD
1981	Donald C. Wharton, MD
1982	Anita Johnson, MD
1983	Stephen J. Atsaves, MD
1984	Anita Johnson, MD
1985	Nelson D. Sanchez, MD
1986	Joseph Danon, MD
1987	Michael R. Treister, MD
1988	Thomas Malvar, MD
1989	Yukhol Lertsburapa, MD
1990	Houshang Farahvar, MD
1991	Zahurul Huq, MD
1992	John P. Monteverde, MD
1993	Nam S. Huh, MD
1994	John C. Przypyszny, MD
1995	Mary L. Klodnycky, MD (President-Elect)

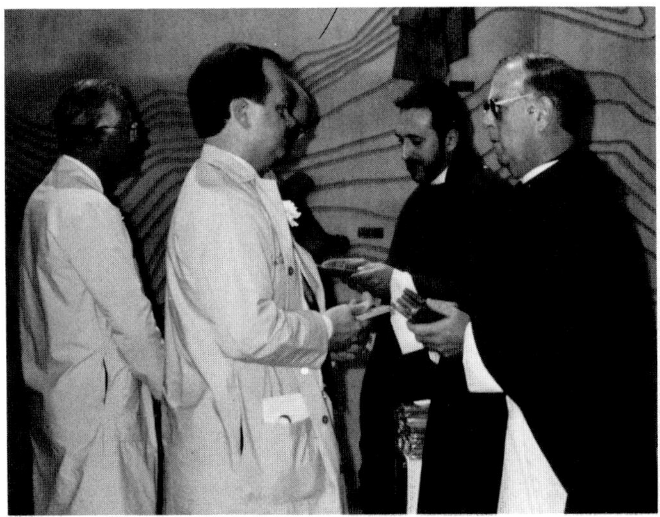

The feast of St. Luke, patron of physicians, is celebrated each year.

OUR PEOPLE

1994 Officers

John C. Przypyszny, MD
President
Mary L. Klodnycky, MD
President-elect
Nam Huh, MD
Immediate Past President
Krish Venugopalan, MD
Secretary
Frank P. Szelag, MD
Treasurer
Maruti S. Bhorade, MD
Staff Representative to AMA
Zahurul Huq, MD
Alternate Staff Representative to AMA

Members at Large:

Edgar A. Borda, MD
Nurer R. Choudhury, MD
Luis Gonzalez-Orozco, MD
Christine S. Hryhorczuk, DDS
Rajogopal Reddy, MD
Mario C. Rosas, MD
Ranchhodlal S. Shah, MD

Medical Staff Department Chairmen

Dentistry
Stephen M. Hashioka, DDS
Lawrence J. Wiatr, DDS, Co-chair

Family Practice
Fernando Cinta, MD
Adolfo M. Llano, MD, Co-chair

General Practice
Mayer Eisenstein, MD
George Dietz, MD, Co-chair

Medicine
Maruti S. Bhorade, MD
Danilo A. Deano, MD, Co-chair

OB/Gynecology
Amalendu Majumsar, MD
Eduardo N. Madamba, MD, Co-chair

Pathology
Mario Velez, MD
Ellen L. Polisky, MD, Co-chair

Pediatrics
Bertha L. Cabrera-Ros, MD
Kalyan B. Sandesara, MD, Co-chair

Psychiatry
Nelson D. Sanchez, MD
Roman T Solecki, MD, Co-chair

Radiology
William V. Mollihan, MD
Ana Stipisic, MD, Co-chair

Surgery
Zahurul Huq, MD
Mohammed N. Siddiqui, MD, Co-chair

Family Practice Residency Program

Adolfo M. Llano, MD
Director

Assistant Directors:
Jean E. Bourand, MD
George Dietz, MD
Boguslaw Nikodem, MD
Mario C. Rosas, MD
Joseph W. Sadowski, MD
Frank P. Szelag, MD

Podiatric Surgical Residency Program

Thomas Kiely, DPM
Director

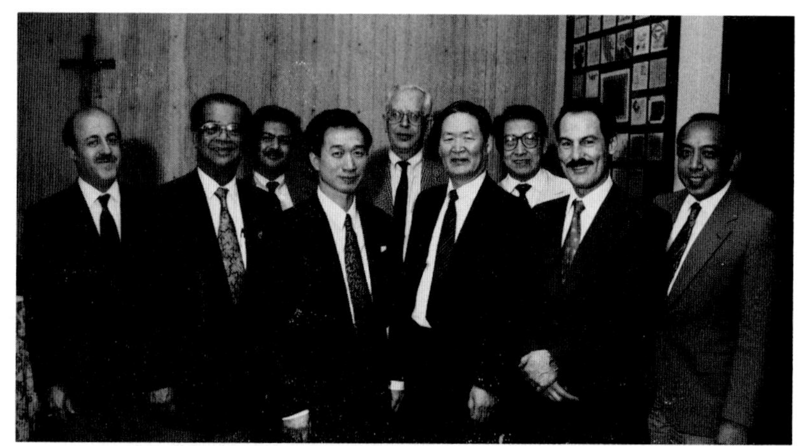

A group of Saint Mary's physicians—left to right: Dr. Houshang Farahvar, Dr. Zahurul Huq, Dr. Mohammed Siddiqui, Dr. John Monteverde, Dr. John Skuza, Dr. Nam Huh, Dr. Yukhol Lertsburapa, Dr. Mouhammad Tarsha and Dr. Danilo Deano

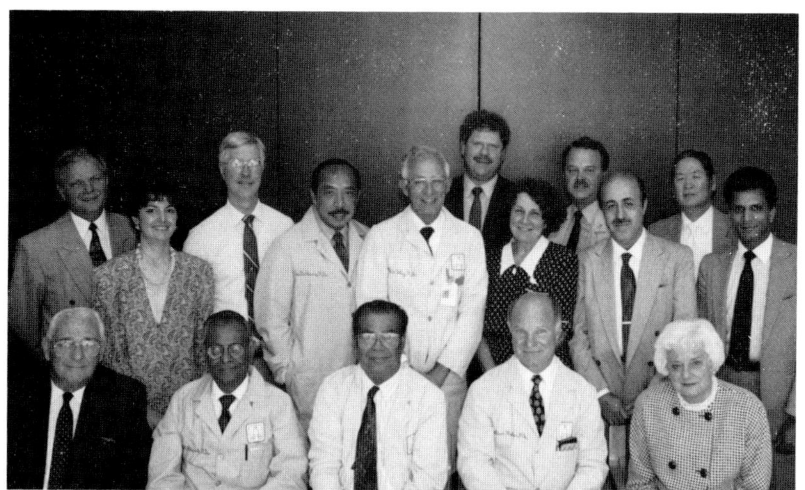

The 1993 Fall Benefit Committee was responsible for the most successful Fall Benefit in its 25-year history. Top row, left to right are: Walter Block, fund development; Phyllis Pavese, public relations; Dr. Gerald Sunko, benefit co-chairman; Dr. Danilo Deano; Dr. Mario Velez; Dr. Michael Treister; Dr. Mary Klodnycky; Dr. Bruce Becker; Dr. Houshang Farahvar; Dr. Nam Huh; Dr. Krish Venugopalan. Bottom row, left to right are: Dr. Salvatore Motto; Dr. Maruti Bhorade; Dr. Zahurul Huq; Dr. William Mollihan, benefit chairman; Irene Allman, administration.

Chairpersons of the Annual Medical Staff Fall Benefit

1969 John E. Meyenberg, MD
The Drake Hotel

1970 Salvatore A. Motto, MD
The Continental Plaza Hotel

1971 Joseph J. Strzyz, MD
McCormick Place

1972 Anthony B. Vacante, MD
The Conrad Hilton Hotel

1973 Jorge R. Tovar, MD
The Conrad Hilton Hotel

1974 Conrad Wiet, MD
The Conrad Hilton Hotel

1975 Procopio U. Yanong, MD
McCormick Place

1976 Donald C. Wharton, MD
The Ritz-Carlton Chicago

1977 Stephen J. Atsaves, MD
The Hyatt Regency Chicago

1978 Bruce P. Zummo, MD
The Hyatt Regency Chicago

1979 Robert Swastek, MD
The Hyatt Regency Chicago

1980 Bruno Valadka, MD
The Continental Plaza Hotel

1981 Hugo R. Velarde, MD
The Hyatt Regency Chicago

1982 Michael R. Treister, MD
The Hyatt Regency Chicago

1983 Julio Ferrer, MD
The Chicago O'Hare Marriott Hotel

1984 Zahurul Huq, MD
The Chicago Marriott Hotel

1985 Ana Stipisic, MD
The Chicago Hilton and Towers

1986 Nelson D. Sanchez, MD
The Chicago Marriott Hotel

1987 James J. Elipas, MD
The Field Museum of Natural History

1988 John J. Skuza, MD
The Fairmont Hotel

1989 Mary L. Klodnycky, MD
The Ritz-Carlton Chicago

1990 Gerald C. Sunko, MD
The Fairmont Hotel

1991 Houshang Farahvar, MD
The Fairmont Hotel

1992 Anita Johnson, MD
The Fairmont Hotel

1993 William V. Mollihan, MD
The Fairmont Hotel

1994 John P. Monteverde
The Chicago Marriott Hotel

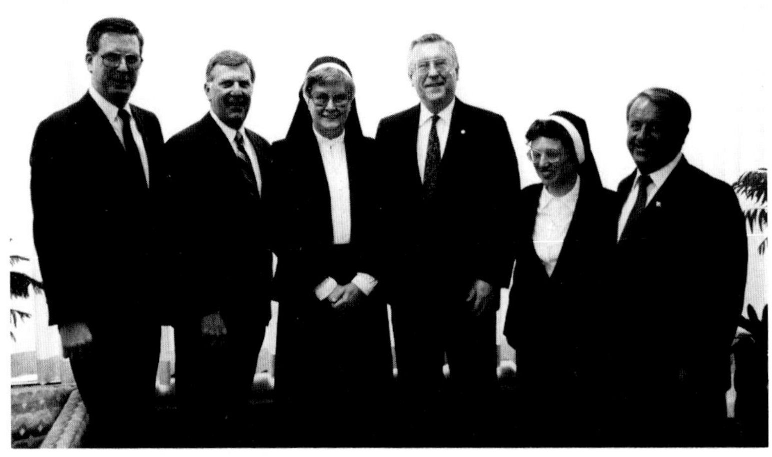

Left to right: Walt Kelly, Mick Donahue, Sister Stella Louise, Eugene Mroz, Sister Kathleen and 1993 Recognition Award Recipient Ed Dykla

The Advisory Board

Presidents

1969-71	John P. Glunz
1972	Irving B. Gerson (Interim)
1972-73	Bernard B. Connolly
1974	Thomas P. O'Donnell
1975-77	Jack C. Leahy
1978-79	Stephen A. Malato
1980-81	William J. Edwards
1982	Henry J. Wozniak
1983-84	Edward J. Allman
1985	E. M. "Mick" Donahue
1986-87	Michael E. Luby
1988-89	E. M. "Mick" Donahue
1990-93	Eugene P. Mroz
1994-	Lawrence J. Ptasinski

1994 Officers

Lawrence J. Ptasinski
President

James Phillips
First Vice President

Larry Sorensen
Second Vice President

Robert M. Fitzgerald
Secretary

Eugene P. Mroz
Immediate Past President

Members

Most Rev. Alfred L. Abramowicz, DD
Edward J. Allman
Allwyn Baptist
William Boyczuk
Rep. Robert Bugielski
Zbigniew Cianciara
Robert Clausen
John A. Cook
E.M. "Mick" Donahue
Edward G. Dykla
Burton Field
Stephen X. Foley, Sr.
Rev. Joseph Glab
Edmund Gronkiewicz
Joseph Katauskas, Jr.
Walter M. Kelly, Jr.
Jack C. Leahy
Michael E. Luby
Honorable Gloria Alitto Majewski
Stephen A. Malato, Sr.
Romuald Matuszczak
Eugene P. Mroz
Mark T. Mroz
Timothy Piech
Andrew Przybylo
James Quinn
Charles F. Scholl
Robert D. Sparr
Gerald C. Sunko, MD
Mitchell Wiet

Honorary Members

Stanley Balzekas, Jr.
King Deets, PhD
Norman Greene
John A. Jeffries
John Lattner
Walter T. McNeely
Raymond Schoessling
Richard Troy
Stanley Wozniak

The Woman's Board

	President	Benefit Chairperson
1971	Irene J. Allman	Rosemary Pavlo
1972	Irene J. Allman	Mary Ann Hackett
1973	Mercedes Foley	Patricia Connolly
1974	Jean Motto	Margaret Bartkowicz
1975	Jean Motto	Eleanor Katauskas
1976	Mary Ann Hackett	Esther Szwaya
1977	Mary Ann Hackett	Elaine Tovar
1978	Elaine Tovar	Vickie Kovacs
1979	Elaine Tovar	Antoinette Manczak
1980	Betty Liberty	Irene J. Allman
1981	Betty Liberty	Eleanor Mirocha
1982	Vickie Kovacs	Barbara Troy
1983	Vickie Kovacs	Jean Motto
1984	Antoinette Manczak	Betty Swastek
1985	Antoinette Manczak	Mary V. Uhrick
1986	Eleanor Mirocha	Janet Zamirowski
1987	Eleanor Mirocha	Ellen Connolly
1988	Eleanor Mirocha	Clare Lemus
1989	Eleanor Mirocha	Barbara Diamond
1990	Lolly Ambers	Eleanor Mirocha
1991	Mary V. Uhrick	Mary Rose Manczak
1992	Mary V. Uhrick	Mary Ann Hackett Betty Liberty
1993	Barbara Diamond	Young Sook Huh
1994	Barbara Diamond	Sylvia Tullo

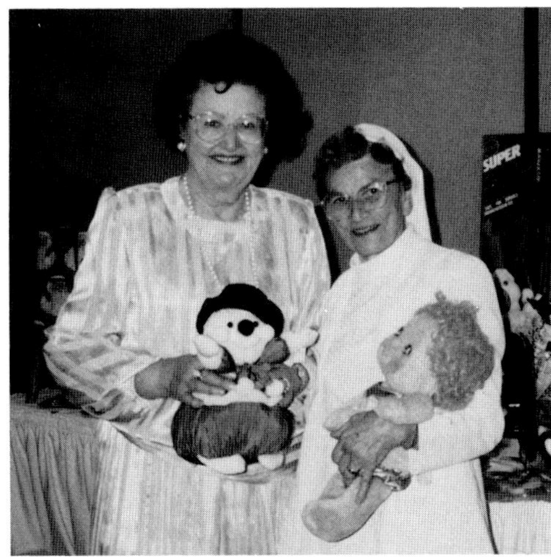

PALS Chairman Jean Motto and Sister Bernadette pose with some of the hundreds of toys donated by Woman's Board members.

1994 Officers

Barbara Diamond
President

Mary Rose Manczak
Vice President

Stella DeFreece
Secretary

Dolores Nielsen
Treasurer

Directors:

Lolly Ambers
Dorothy Schwan
Eleanore Idol
Mary V. Uhrick

Irene J. Allman
Moderator

The Women's Auxiliary

Honorary Presidents

Mrs. Gervaise Pallasch
Mrs. Matthew Uznanski
Felice Walkowicz

Honorary Members

Lillian Jablonski
Mrs. John Novatny
Mrs. Leon Novatny
Nora Rusinek
Mrs. Vincent W. Tondryk

Presidents

1904-05	Mrs. Stephen R. Pietrowicz
1906	Mrs. F.J. Laibe
1907-08	Mrs. Ferdinand Pirnat
1909	Mrs. Stephen R. Pietrowicz
1910	Mrs. George R. Mueller
1911	Mrs. N.R. New
1912	Mrs. Ferdinand Pirnat
1913-14	Mrs. F.H. Westerschulte
1915-16	Mrs. K. Scanlan
1917-18	Mrs. George R. Mueller
1919-20	Mrs. N.R. New
1921-22	Mrs. Leon Grotowski
1923-24	Mrs. Stephen R. Pietrowicz
1925-26	Mrs. Edward Dombrowski
1927-28	Mrs. Leon Grotowski
1929-30	Mrs. Leon Dyniewicz
1931-32	Mrs. Peter R. Mindak
1933	Mrs. Edward Roling
1934-35	Mrs. Edward A. Kirsten
1936	Mrs. B.J. Mix
1937-38	Felice Walkowicz
1939-40	Mrs. Peter J. Doretti
1941-42	Mrs. Leon Grotowski
1943-44	Mrs. Bernard C. Kolter
1945-46	Mrs. Matthew E. Uznanski
1947	Felice Walkowicz
1948-49	Mrs. George R. Mueller
1950-51	Frances Jasinski
1952-53	Mary Casciato
1954-55	Mrs. William C. Jarvis
1956	Sylvia Bruske
1957-58	Mrs. John Luczak
1959-60	Mrs. John Sincere
1961	Sylvia Bruske
1962-63	Mrs. Giles Kirsten
1964-65	Mary Pallasch
1966-68	Jean Tenczar
1969-70	Mrs. Chester Andrzejczak (Strzoda)
1971-73	Mrs. Dominic Chechile
1974-75	Arlene Walczak
1976-80	Helen DeFrancisco
1981-85	Sabina P. Logisz
1986-87	Bernice Zik
1988-92	Lorraine Wilczewski
1993-	Joanne Slowik

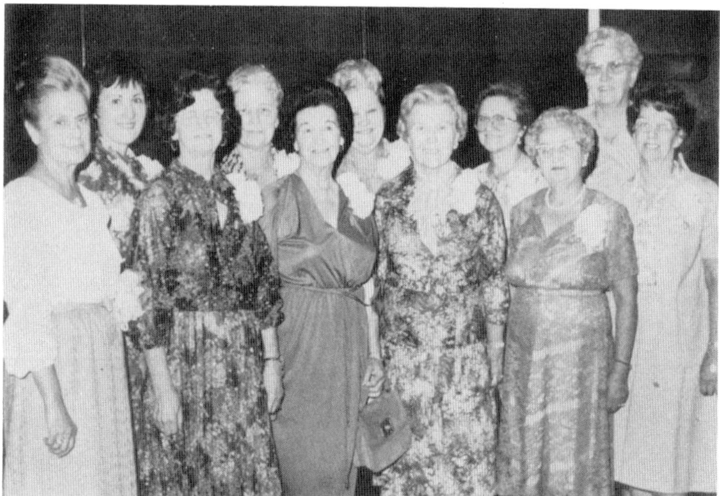

Women's Auxiliary past presidents gathered in 1980. Left to right are: Sabina Logisz, Juliana Strzoda, Mary Palasch, Frances Jasinski, Mary Casciato, Arlene Walczak, Frances Jarvis, Helen Defrancisco, Felice Walkowicz, Sylvia Bruske and Jean Tenczar.

1994 Officers

Joanne Slowik
President

Estelle Sprengel
First Vice President

Sylvia Zimek
Second Vice President

Elaine Annes
Recording Secretary

Lizabeth Stochmal
Financial Secretary

Theresa Fic
Treasurer

Directors:
Helen DeFrancisco
Sabina Logisz
Phyllis Klimek
Robert J. Browne, Jr.
Liaison

Moderators:
Sister Stella Louise, CSFN
Sister M. Valentine, CSFN

OUR PEOPLE

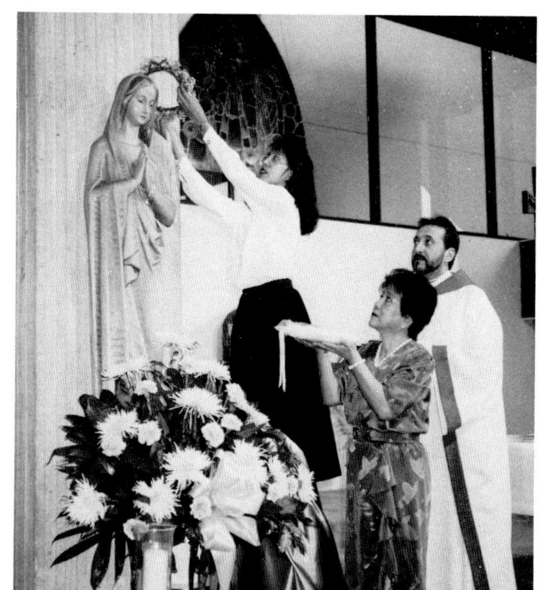

Delmira R. Ibarrientos performs the annual May crowning ceremony in the hospital chapel, assisted by Natividad R. Loleng. Both employees work in patient accounting services. Father John Kobus is at right.

Corporate Officers

Sister Stella Louise, CSFN, FACHE
President and Chief Executive Officer

Thomas O. Meirink
Executive Vice President, Hospital Operations

Kenneth A. Kautzer
Senior Vice President, Finance, and Treasurer

Bruce C. Becker II, MD
Vice President, Medical Affairs, Education and Research

C. Wayne Hamilton
Vice President, Corporate Development and Marketing

Corporate and Administrative Staff

Irene J. Allman, RN
Vice President, Clinical Services

Janie L. Campbell, PhD, RN
Vice President, Patient Services

Bernard H. Henry
Vice President, Human Resources

Linda Kennedy
Vice President, Continuous Quality Improvement

Robert J. Konkel
Vice President, Financial Services

William S. Strzoda
Vice President, Hospital Support Services

Joseph L. Boton
Assistant Administrator, Marketing and Communications

Patrick Burke
Assistant Administrator, Medical Support and Managed Care

Sister Kathleen Ann, CSFN
Assistant Administrator, Continuing Care

Walter F. Block
Director, Fund Development

Lisa Maher
Assistant to the President/Risk Manager and Government Relations

Kasha Cianciara
Public Relations Specialist

Mary Daly
Fund Development Associate

Phyllis Pavese
Director, Creative Services

Victor Villalobos
Community Relations Specialist

Pastoral Care Staff

Father John Kobus, Director
Father Lawrence Henry
Father Paul Liwanag
Sister M. Blanche, CSFN

Management Staff

Cardiology
John Sedivy

Emergency Department
Beverly Weaver, RN

Facilities Engineering and Maintenance
Richard L. Dusing Jr.

Family Practice Center/Outpatient Services/JOBMED
Angela Openlander, RN

Finance Department
Bob Cech

Food and Nutrition Services
Wardley Birkett, RD

Housekeeping
Maria N. Roman

Information Management
Jorge S. Cerda

Land and Facilities Development
Andrew Mylniczenko

Materials Management
Edward Hogan

Medical Education
Mary Roper

Medical Library
Olivia Fistrovic

Medical Records
Jeanette Kebisek

Mental Health Center
Michael S. Pelletier

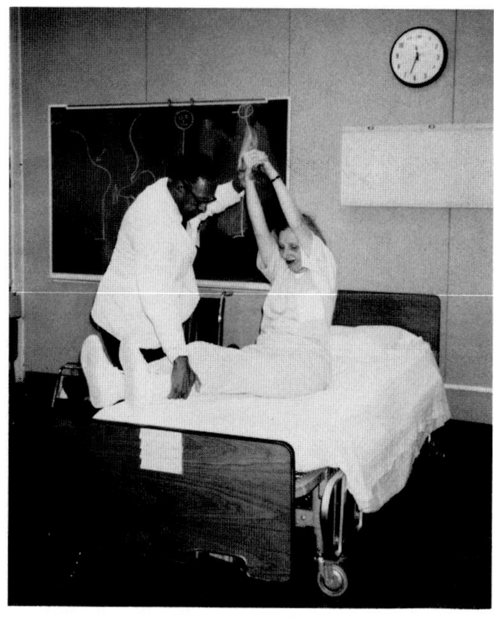

Wendell Venerable, Physical/Occupational Therapy Director, is assisted in a demonstration by Angela Openlander, Director of Medishare and Family

Nursing—Obstetrics/Women's Services
Margaret Cincotta, RN

Nursing—Medical/Surgical/Pediatrics/Respiratory Care
Elsa Goyma, RN

Nursing—Operative Units
Rose Krogh, RN

Nursing—Organization Standards and Education
Sister M. Antonia, CSFN, RN, MSN

Occupational Therapy/Physical Medicine
Wendell Venerable

Pathology Laboratories
John T. Preston, PhD

Patient Financial Services
Lilia Comendador

Pharmaceutical Services
William T. Lee, RPh

Quality Improvement
Sherri Kohnen, RN, BSN

Radiology
William Plos, RT

Respiratory Therapy
Louise Lewis

Security/Transportation
George Mizia
Social Work
Kathy Driscoll

Telecommunications
Laura Webb

Volunteer Services
Robert J. Browne Jr.

Marketing Coordinators

Ambulatory Surgery/Orthopedics
Thomas Aitken

Cardiology
Joseph O'Donnell, MS

Mental Health
Dan Ortego

Oncology/Diabetes
Sylvia Watts

Head Nurses

Coronary Care Unit/Intensive Care Unit
Cecilia Beauprie, RN

2nd Floor—Adult Psychiatry
Manuel Mercado, RN

5th Floor—OB/Gyne
Ellen Zakrzewski, RN
Assistant—Sophia Kass, RN

6th Floor—Pediatrics/Orthopedics/Rehabilitation
Marlene McGann, RN
Assistant—Fran Teti-Teal, RN

7th Floor—Telemetry Nursing
Mary Lopez, RN

9th Floor—Ambulatory Surgery/Same DayAdmission
Pat Graham, RN

11th Floor—Oncology/Hematology
Erika Skomoroch, RN

12th Floor—Medical/Diabetic
Sonya Tan-Sandiego, RN

14th Floor—Medical/Surgical
Molly Lobo, RN

15th Floor—Adolescent Psychiatry
Efrem Sarmiento, RN

16th Floor—Adult Psychiatry
Soyoun Choi, RN

1994 Medical Staff Members

Frida R. Abrahamian, MD
Sikander Adeni, MD
Brojendra Agarwala, MD
Jorge N. Aguayo, MD
Ashraf Ahmed, MD
Safia S. Ahmed, MD
Harpinder Ajmani, MD
Otto Aldana, MD
Jorge A. Aliaga, MD
Raquel Alvarez, MD
Hong-Chan An, MD
Satyavathi Anne, MD
Frank O. Apantaku, MD
Lina L. Aquino, MD
Mohammed Araghi, DDS
Vijay Arekapudi, MD
Ada Arias, MD
Solomon Aronson, MD
Stephen J. Atsaves, DDS
Mila R. Bacalla, MD
Yaroslaw Bandura, MD
Henryk Baraniewski, MD
Bruce C. Becker II, MD
Nora F. Beltran, MD
Julio N. Berjon, MD
Krystyna H. Berry, MD
Maruti S. Bhorade, MD
Robin B. Blakkolb, DDS
Zofia Bochacki, MD
Krystyna Bochinska, MD
Leo R. Boler Jr., MD
Edgar A. Borda, MD
Jean E. Bourand, MD
Paul F. Brezinski, DPM
Walter Brodech, MD
Maria I. Brown, DO
Thomas J. Burke, MD
Bertha L. Cabrera-Ros, MD
Emile Cambry, MD
Adalberto Campo, MD
Elmer A. Carasig, MD
Rafael P. Carreira, MD
Carmelita T. Carriaga, MD
James M. Caruso, MD
Samuel Castillo, MD
Walter Cebulski, MD
Chung K. Chen, MD
Henry K. Chen, MD
Nurer R. Choudhury, MD
Chris N. Choukas, DDS
Shabbir Chowdhry, MD
David Chua, MD
Sam M. Ciccarelli, DDS
Fernando Cinta, MD
Mary J. Cipriani, MD
Asuncion J. Claveria, MD
Edward A. Cohen, MD
Philip G. Coleman, MD
Theodore C. Compall, MD
John V. Courtney, MD
Beata Danek, MD
Joseph Danon, MD
Antonio G. DeLeon, MD
Danilo A. Deano, MD
Jose B. Delfin, MD
Alfonso Diaz, MD
George Dietz, MD
Morteza M. Dini, MD
Ester C. Dionisio, MD
Aleksy Dobradin, MD
Ashokkumar M. Doshi, MD
Thomas C. Draghi, MD
Michael Earley, MD
Mayer Eisenstein, MD
James J. Elipas, DPM
Rodrigo F. Endara, MD
Manuel M. Escalona Jr, MD
Pilarita Espinosa, MD
Robert J. Familaro, DDS
Houshang Farahvar, MD
Anna M. Farkas, MD

James Feinberg, MD
Jose Fernandez, MD
Julio C. Ferrer, MD
Michael J. Fisher, MD
John Flanagan, DPM
Jean Flood, MD
M. Michael Forutan, MD
Leon J. Frazin, MD
John A. Gall, MD
Mrugendra M. Gandhi, MD
Vikram H. Gandhi, MD
Vivek Ghai, MD
Joseph M. Giannini, DPM
Michael W. Giannini, MD
Janice L. Gilden, MD
Juliette J. Giner, MD
Cai Glushak, MD
Hilda Goldbarg, MD
Carlos A. Gomez, MD
Benigno J. Gonzalez, MD
Luis Gonzalez-Orozco, MD
Joseph L. Graziano, MD
Andrew J. Griffin, MD
Eugenia M. Grochowska, MD
Francisco A. Gutierrez, MD
Hamid A. Hai, MD
Long K. Han, MD
Stephen M. Hashioka, DDS
Farhana Hassan, MD
Ernst J. Holland, MD
Ronald Holt, MD
Ok R. Hong, MD
Christine S. Hryhorczuk, DDS
Nam S. Huh, MD
Zahurul Huq, MD
Michal Hytros, MD
Eddie C. Inocencio, MD
Orest Jachtorowycz, MD
Manohar Jasuja, MD
Carlito C. Javier, MD
Bangalore N. Jayaram, MD
Krystyna B. Jedrychowska, MD
Anita Johnson, MD
Nalinaksha V. Joshi, MD
Lilliana Jovanovic, MD
Bozena B. Jurek, MD
Peter Jurek, MD
Mitchell V. Kaminski Jr., MD
M. Orhan Kaymakcalan, MD
Rajeev Khanna, MD
Thomas Kiely, DPM
Ann M. Kieran, MD
Chang S. Kim, MD
Choong G. Kim, MD
Tong S. Kim, MD
Felismeno G. Kintanar, MD
Mary L. Klodnycky, MD
Philip J. Konecny, MD
Kevin J. Kozie, DPM
Lee J. Kozie, DPM
Leonard I. Kranzler, MD
David P. Kumamoto, DDS
Peter Kurko, MD
Pawel K. Kwiecinski, MD
Eduardo J. Ladlad, MD
Julio Lara-Valle, MD
Seung S. Lee, MD
Yukhol Lertsburapa, MD
Chung-Yuan Lin, MD
Ramon R. Lipardo, MD
Adolfo M. Llano, MD
Michel Louvain, MD
Prasert Luangkesorn, MD
Eduardo N. Madamba, MD
M. Munir Maghrabi, DPM
Amalendu Majumdar, MD
Mansour V. Makhlouf, MD
Thomas Malvar, MD
Francisco B. Mariano, MD
Bayoan C. Mateo, MD
Mary J. McCabe, MD
Luis E. Mendoza, DPM
Cesar Menendez, MD
Alvaro Mercado, MD
Cynthia M. Mercado, DPM
Kent Mercado, DPM
Orlando A. Mercado, DPM
Ramiro Mercado, MD
John E. Meyenberg, MD
James A. Meyer, MD
Vahed Mirafzali, MD
William V. Mollihan, MD
John P. Monteverde, MD
Louis Morales, DPM
Arnold S. Morof, DDS
Salvatore A. Motto, MD
Henry Munez, MD
Rafaela Munoz-Ulrich, MD
Chitra V. Nadimpalli, MD
Antonio Navarrete, MD
Herman J. Neal, MD
Boguslaw Nikodem, MD
Kyung Noh, MD
Waldemar Nowak, MD
Ausencio Nunez, MD
Myo Nwe, MD
Donal O'Sullivan, MD
Miguel Ochoa, MD
Philip D. Ogden, MD
Neftali Otero, MD
Eniola A. Owi, MD
Edwin V. Palileo, MD
G. Velayudha Paniker, MD
Dilipkumar C. Parikh, MD
Chung D. Park, MD
Amritbhai P. Patel, MD
Chandulal M. Patel, MD
Hemant R. Patel, MD
Natu R. Patel, MD
Virendra M. Patel, MD
Walter A. Pedemonte, MD
Raymond J. Pellicore, MD
Anthony Perez, DPM
Albert P. Pietrasik, MD
Olga A. Pietruk, MD
Ellen L. Polisky, MD
Gopal K. Popli, MD
Thomas K. Poulakidas, DDS
John C. Przypyszny, MD
Raghu Ramadurai, MD
Ramesh P. Rao, MD
Sripathy U. Rao, MD
Biswamay Ray, MD
Rajagopal Reddy, MD
Jader Reis, MD
Christos K. Rekkas, MD
Dominick S. Renga, MD
Peter D. Roberson, DDS
Jesus C. Rodenas, MD
Mario C. Rosas, MD
Orest P. Rywak, MD
Seshadri Sadagopan, MD
Joseph W. Sadowski, MD
Julita Sadowski, MD

Franklin B. Saksena, MD
Nelson D. Sanchez, MD
Kalyan B. Sandesara, MD
Anthony R. Sapienza, MD
Leslie Schaffer, MD
Paul Schattauer, MD
Howard O. Schechter, MD
Maria Serratto-Benvenuto, MD
Ranchhodlal S. Shah, MD
Bansi D. Sharma, MD
Mohammed N. Siddiqui, MD
Shanti Siddiqui, MD
Margaret M. Sierantowicz, MD
Anthony N. Silvetti, MD
Lafayette Singleton Jr., MD
Mohammad Sirajullah, MD
John J. Skuza, MD
Hilliard E. Slavick, MD
Wojciech Slodowy, MD
Apollo C. Solecki, MD
Roman T. Solecki, MD
Robert M. Sommerfeld, DDS
George R. Sosenko, MD
Lisa A. Spatz, MD
Christiane E. Stahl, MD
Augustyn Stec, MD
Kenneth L. Stein, MD
Ana Stipisic, MD
Aleksandra A. Stobnicki, MD
Alan Summers, MD
Borys A. Sumyk, MD
Gerald C. Sunko, MD
Robert T. Swastek, MD
Frank P. Szelag, MD
Christine Szymik, MD
Chee-Ken Tan, MD
Waldemar Taraszkiewicz, MD
Mouhammad F. Tarsha, MD
Thana Tarsha, MD
Ben J. Tatarowicz, MD
Constantine J. Tatooles, MD
Alan J. Tenczar, DPM
Theodore R. Tenczar, MD
John Thachil, MD
Korathu Thomas, MD
Jorge R. Tovar, MD
Michael R. Treister, MD
Victor M. Uribe, MD
Bruno Valadka, MD
Venkata S. Vedam, MD
Hugo R. Velarde, MD
Mario Velez, MD
Krish Venugopalan, MD
Boris A. Vern, MD
Remegio M. Vilbar, MD
Flordeliza G. Villafuerte, MD
Roger Villalba, MD
Jon Waldman, MD
Franchot H.C. Wang, MD
Donald C. Wharton, MD
Lawrence J. Wiatr, DDS
Elizabeth T. Wieckiewicz, MD
Gary G. Wiesman, MD
Jozef Wilk, MD
Lucjan Witkowski, MD
Ruth M. Yanagi, MD
Jose U. Yanong, MD
Jovita U. Yanong, MD
Pio U. Yanong, MD
Procopio U. Yanong, MD
Wesley Y. Yapor, MD
Robert F. Yario, MD
Julio C. Yarzagaray, MD
Sharukin Yelda, MD
Steven F. Yellen, MD
Hazim Y. Zakko, MD
Richard W. Zalar, MD
Helio C. Zapata, MD
Javier Zavaleta, MD
Mark Zumhagen, MD
Bruce P. Zummo, MD

Saint Mary of Nazareth Hospital Center
Affiliations and Accreditations

Accredited by:

- The Joint Commission on Accreditation of Healthcare Organizations
- The Council of Medical Education and Hospitals
- The American Medical Association
- The United States Department of Health and Human Services
- The Department of Public Aid
- The Chicago Board of Health
- The Council on Podiatric Medical Education of the American Podiatric Medical Association
- The Accreditation Council for Graduate Medical Education of the AMA for Family Practice Residency, and an approved site for Medical Clerkships in Community and Family Medicine by Loyola University Stritch School of Medicine

Licensed by:

- The State of Illinois
- The City of Chicago

A member of:

- The Catholic Health Association
- The American Hospital Association
- The Illinois Catholic Hospital Association
- The Illinois Hospital Association
- The Catholic Health Alliance of Metropolitan Chicago
- Metropolitan Chicago Healthcare Council
- The Blue Cross Plan for Hospital Care
- The American Management Association
- The Conference of Teaching Hospitals

Prayer of Hospitality

(This prayer appears at all entrances to Saint Mary of Nazareth Hospital Center.)

Sacred is this threshold of our hospital and holy is this door. This is the meeting place of friend, neighbor and stranger. May it be a bridge for our comings and goings. Whenever we stand within its sacred circle, may our eyes be granted new vision so that we can see in friend or stranger the God of ten thousand disguises.

May this threshold be a sacred place where we come to celebrate the sacrament of hospitality. May the spirits of evil never cross this threshold and may the name of the All Holy One protect our hospital from harm. May God's angels stand guard to the right and left of this opening to grace our comings and goings.

May we who work in this hospital guard the sacredness of this doorway. May our hearts be always alert to the dangers of falseness and pretense as we greet those who come to our door. Let our affection be graced with honesty and reverence and the oil of our truth burn in the lamp of our eyes. Help us to remember that our ancestors were strangers and exiled in Egypt, that Joseph and Mary came knocking at a door like this, weary and in search of kindness. May we receive all at this door as godly guests.

May the blessings of God and the peace and grace of the All Holy One surround this threshold and rest upon all who shall pass across it. Amen.